Fast Facts

for the Family Medicine Board Review

D1452058

Fast Facts

for the Family Medicine Board Review

Frank J. Domino, MD

Professor and Director of Predoctoral Education
Department of Family Medicine and Community Health
University of Massachusetts Medical School
Worcester, Massachusetts

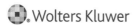 Wolters Kluwer

Philadelphia · Baltimore · New York · London
Buenos Aires · Hong Kong · Sydney · Tokyo

Acquisitions Editor: Rebecca Gaertner
Senior Developmental Editor: Kristina Oberle
Editorial Coordinator: Emily Buccieri
Marketing Manager: Rachel Mante Leung
Production Project Manager: Bridgett Dougherty
Design Coordinator: Holly McLaughlin
Manufacturing Coordinator: Beth Welsh
Prepress Vendor: S4Carlisle Publishing Services

9 8 7 6 5 4 3 2 1

Printed in China

Library of Congress Cataloging-in-Publication Data

Names: Domino, Frank J., author.
Title: Fast facts for the family medicine board review / Frank J. Domino.
Description: Philadelphia : Wolters Kluwer Heath, [2017] | Includes index.
Identifiers: LCCN 2017012816 | ISBN 9781496370891
Subjects: | MESH: Family Practice | Examination Questions
Classification: LCC R834.5 | NLM WB 18.2 | DDC 610.76—dc23
    LC record available at https://lccn.loc.gov/2017012816

LWW.com

Preface

"Real knowledge is to know the extent of one's ignorance"
Confucius

I was a horrible test taker. Ask my former classmates. Despite a strong knowledge base and reasonable patient interaction skills, my arch nemesis was the multiple choice test. I share this fact with my students and residents to remind them they are far more than a score. Yet, the American Board of Family Medicine requires we pass an initial exam to become board certified, and then repeat that daylong experience every 10 years or so.

There are two important components to success on medical board exams. Confidence in your test-taking skill is paramount, as I learned the hard way. And a strong, current, and accessible knowledgebase. This book hopes to focus on the latter. Its goal is to give you brief snippets of the clinical knowledge you need to succeed as a family physician. Its format is to allow you to first quickly read its content and then practice testing your knowledge. The content covers a broad scope and is directed to the most important components of disease and treatment. To help with the knowledgebase, I have helped develop this book.

Frank J. Domino, MD

Acknowledgments

Like any endeavor, this is more the work of many, with me just leading the way. Chelsea Harris, MD, Avinash Sridhar, MD, and Diana Ong, MD, read and helped shape the content. I am in their debt and offer my thanks. Robert Baldor, MD, author and editor of Baldor's Family Medicine Board Review text provided his wonderful mentorship while sharing content suggestions and reflections and is deeply responsible in making this book a reality. I thank Rebecca Gaertner and Kristina Oberle from Wolters Kluwer; they were patient, helpful, and supportive through this process; this would not be in your hands without their expertise and guidance.

Finally, I must thank all who helped me survive the horror of my test-taking days. This nightmare ended for me a few years back, when I realized that standardized tests are just another skill to be learned. Looking back, those who supported me through my personal hell include Mark Quirk, EdD, Drew Grimes, MD, and Robert Smith, DO, and many physician colleagues. But mostly it was my family, from my parents, Angela and Frank Domino, and brother, John Domino, who somehow saw beneath my poor test scores someone who could succeed, and my wife, Sylvia, and daughter, Molly, who had my back when I needed it the most.

Frank J. Domino, MD

American Board of Family Medicine Examination Structure

The goal of the ABFM's examination is for family physicians to demonstrate "cognitive expertise." Family medicine was one of the first specialties to require repeated demonstration of this expertise and supports our position as a specialty, where keeping current with the delivery of healthcare is a priority.

The content of the 2017 exam (what the ABFM calls its "Blueprint") is as follows:

Respiratory 11%
Cardiovascular 10%
Musculoskeletal 10%
Nonspecific 8%
Endocrine 7%
Gastrointestinal 6%
Psychogenic 6%
Integumentary 5%
Population-based care 4% (biostatistics/ epidemiology, evidence-based medicine, prevention, health policy/legal issues, bioterrorism, quality improvement, and geographic/urban/rural issues)
Patient-based systems 4% (clinical decision making, doctor-patient interaction, family and cultural issues, ethics, palliative care, and end-of-life care)
Neurologic 3%
Nephrologic 3%
Hematologic/Immune 3%
Reproductive—Female 3%
Special Sensory 2%
Reproductive—Male 1%

In 2017, our exam was shortened to 320 questions from 370 questions. There are 4 sections of 80 questions each. The module you select will have 40 questions and the remainder of the exam will be general family medicine questions.

The exam requires the tester to choose one specialty area to demonstrate extra knowledge. In past years, they required two. These include ambulatory family medicine, child and adolescent care, geriatrics, women's health, maternity care, emergent/urgent care, hospital medicine, and sports medicine.

For a full description of the exam and its process, head to the ABFM website: https://www.theabfm.org/moc/cognitive.aspx

. . .

The Skill and Art of Test Taking

The goal of the ABFM is to have you demonstrate your competency as a family physician. It is not to trick you or "weed out" some subset. This is very different than your licensing examinations of medical school. With this in mind, remember, they want you to succeed.

Knowing this, there are a number of simple guidelines you can apply to your test taking to help you pass.

1. Which to do: read the question or answer first. No data support one method as better than another. So do what you feel fits your style; most of us benefit from reading the entire question first.
2. Read the **entire** question. This is the most common test-taking error. Do not skim the words in the question, because...
3. The ANSWER is always in the question. The question writers give you hints all through the question to direct you to the correct answer (remember, they want you to succeed). Remember, when you hear hoof beats, do not think zebras. If the question tells you about a patient who is recovering from a stroke who develops fatigue and confusion, whose serum sodium is low and urinary osmolality is high, the answer is likely SIADH and NOT something even more rare.
4. Read all of the answers. As you go through them, eliminate those that are incorrect. Do not stop when you find the answer you think is correct.
5. Ignore "if" answers. These answers are called distractors. If you have to use the word "if" before an answer, then it is wrong. In pressured situations, they are effective at confusing your thoughts. "If the patient was an alcoholic, their sodium could be low." No "if."
6. The answer is the NEXT STEP. The correct answer to any question is for you to address the most pressing issue. If the patient has a fever and a change in mental status, initiating treatment, not getting an MRI or CT, is the next step.
7. When you have no idea, use partial knowledge. Look in the question and answers for things you know, eliminate answers you believe are incorrect, choose from the one that remains, and never look back. Because...
8. Never change an answer... unless some future question reminds you of a correct answer in a former question. But this is very rare. So, once you choose an answer, unless you are certain, never change.
9. Knowledge deficit. This means you do not know some content. However, you no longer have to worry about this issue, as you now have all of the answers in your hands. But if you find a question that stumps you, just read the answers. Choose one, and quickly move on.

Smile! You now have all of the skills and knowledge to succeed at the American Board of Family Medicine certification examination. Look at this task as a learning experience. Find those things you did not know and gladly add them to your thinking. And thank you for being a Family Physician. It is the best job in the world.

Frank J. Domino, M.D.

Contents

CHAPTER
1 Pediatrics

1. Phototherapy for hyperbilirubinemia should be initiated in a newborn at 35 or more weeks of gestation when total serum bilirubin (TSB) is

29–48 hours (2 days) at >15 mg/dL
49–72 hours (3 days) at >18 mg/dL
72 hours (> 3 days) at >20 mg/dL
Or >5 mg/dL/day

---

2. A premature infant develops abdominal distention and is very ill after initiation of feeding. What is the greatest concern?

Necrotizing enterocolitis (NEC): a diffuse necrotic injury to the bowel, which can result in perforation or subserosal collections of gas

---

3. Juvenile idiopathic arthritis (formerly known as juvenile rheumatoid arthritis) is associated with what eye finding?

Uveitis

---

4. Strep throat modified Centor criteria include what clinical findings?

- Age (5–15 years)
- Tonsillar exudates
- Tender, enlarged (1 cm) anterior cervical lymph nodes (posterior chain nodes imply viral illness, most commonly mononucleosis)
- Fever
- Absence of cough and rhinorrhea

---

5. What is the most common cause of amblyopia (decreased vision in one or both eyes due to abnormal development of vision in infancy or childhood)?

Strabismus (turn of the eye)

---

6. Who develops NEC?	NEC is most commonly seen in premature infants in the first 3 weeks of life, but 10% of those who develop NEC are born at term.
7. Nasal polyps are associated with what pediatric chronic pulmonary condition?	Cystic fibrosis
8. A previously continent 6-year-old male has repeated stool soiling of his underwear. What condition needs to be addressed?	Constipation; encopresis is defined as repeated unintentional soiling of underwear and is commonly associated with functional constipation with severe stool retention and subsequent overflow incontinence.
9. What is the most likely etiology of proteinuria in children?	Transient proteinuria that can be caused by fever, exercise, seizures, and/or hypovolemia Orthostatic (postural) hypotension is a common cause of proteinuria in children, where protein excretion can be high with standing and return to normal when supine.
10. What are the clinical features of a cephalohematoma?	Swelling of the scalp, with edema located below the periosteum of the skull that does not cross suture lines; it is caused by rupture of vessels during delivery.
11. How is pediatric encopresis treated?	Initial fecal disimpaction with oral polyethylene glycol (PEG-3 350 (0.75 mg/kg/24 h) and behavioral modification (child to sit on toilet for defined amount of time (1 min/year of age to a maximum of 10 minutes) 1–2 times per day (ideally after a meal) and perform a Valsalva maneuver (blow into a pinwheel or a balloon to try to make them bear down). Should use a sticker/star chart to reward success. Diet should include high fiber and water, and elimination of all highly processed foods and sweetened foods and drinks.

12. What is the difference between primary and secondary enuresis?	Primary nocturnal enuresis (NE) is most common; child/adult who has never established urinary continence on consecutive nights for a period of $\geq$6 months; secondary NE: resumption of enuresis after at least 6 months of urinary continence
13. What is the natural course of a cephalohematoma?	Most will resolve by themselves in a few weeks Complications include hyperbilirubinemia, calcification, infection
14. What is caput succedaneum?	Swelling of the scalp, edema is located above the periosteum of the skull; findings can cross suture lines, and may or may not be bloody.
15. What is a subgaleal hemorrhage?	Swelling is over the entire scalp, feels boggy and fluctuant. Edema is located between the periosteum of the skull and the aponeurosis. Edema can cross the suture line; is bloody and caused by shearing of emissary veins during delivery Risk of massive blood loss and mortality (12%–14%).
16. What is Erb palsy?	"Waiter's tip;" Upper brachial plexus injury due to injury during birth leaving the arm extended and hand palmar flexed. Examine for clavicular fracture.
17. What is the most common cause of secondary enuresis?	Situational stress: family stress, depression, anxiety, social phobias, conduct disorder, hyperkinetic syndrome, internalizing disorders
18. What is Klumpke palsy?	When a paralysis of the hand and wrist results in a claw hand; often with Horner syndrome (miosis, ptosis, anhidrosis)
19. What are the physical exam findings of phimosis?	The inability to retract foreskin

20. What is the common term for and clinical course of genu varum?	Bow-legged; usually resolves between 18–24 months.
21. What is the common term for and clinical course of genu valgus?	Knock knees; usually resolves before age 10. Physiologic genu valgus will see improvement over time, but pathologic valgus will typically worsen after age 4.
22. What are the physical exam findings and clinical course of talipes equinovarus?	Clubfoot. Will not self-correct and patient should be referred to an orthopedic specialist. Initial management includes manipulation and stretching of the foot.
23. What are the physical exam findings and clinical course of metatarsus adductus?	The forefoot turns toward midline. Most will self-correct by age 2.
24. What is transient tachypnea of the newborn?	Pulmonary edema in the newborn caused by delayed clearance and resorption of fetal lung fluid. More often seen in premature babies and babies born with cesarean sections. TTN often resolves in the first 48 hours of life.
25. What are the common treatments for primary enuresis?	Simple behavioral interventions: (e.g., scheduled wakening, positive reinforcement, bladder training, diet changes). Encourage reduction of liquids intake in the hours prior to sleep; regular bedtime with full night's sleep, scheduled voiding before bed, nightlights to light the way to the bathroom, reward system for dry nights. If all these fail, consider use of bed alarms or desmopressin (DDAVP).
26. What are clinical features of transient tachypnea of the newborn?	Tachypnea (> 60 minutes) within the first 2 hours of delivery, which is self-limiting, and care is supportive.
27. What speed is the acceptable newborn heart rate?	120–160 beats/min

28. What is the normal newborn respiratory rate?	30–60 breaths/min.
29. What are the common treatments for secondary enuresis?	Address stressors at home and at school. If constipation, use of PEG-3550. Behavioral interventions similar to primary enuresis (limiting late night liquids, bedtime toileting, etc.).
30. In infants, what is the most common cancer?	Neuroblastoma
31. What genetic condition is associated with meconium ileus in the newborn?	Cystic fibrosis
32. A 12-month child who is less than 2 standard deviations from the mean for weight or whose weight for chronologic age is less than the 5th percentile has what condition?	Failure to thrive
33. What pediatric condition is associated with prolonged fever, a non-exudative conjunctivitis, fissured lips, strawberry tongue, cervical adenopathy, and an erythematous polymorphous rash?	Kawasaki disease
34. What is the female athlete triad?	Clinical syndrome of low energy availability (eating disorder +/- exercise expenditure greater than calories consumed), menstrual dysfunction (commonly amenorrhea due to low estrogen state), and low bone mineral density
35. Prolonged jaundice in a newborn is suggestive of	Biliary atresia

36. How can you differentiate between slipped capital femoral epiphysis (SCFE) and Legg–Calve–Perthes disease?

By age. Legg–Calvé–Perthes (necrosis of femoral head): 4–10 years of age; SCFE adolescent boys over the age of 10 years. The two conditions have similar features, and include antalgic gait, resistance to internal rotation, and insidious onset.

37. Erythema toxicum is commonly known as

Newborn acne

38. In newborns, what time period should birth weight be regained?

2 weeks

39. What are likely diagnoses if no passage of meconium occurs within 24 hours of birth?

Imperforate anus, Hirshsprung disease, or cystic fibrosis

40. In exclusively breastfed infants, what is the only additional supplementation recommended?

Vitamin D supplementation of 400 IU/day

41. What is a severe complication associated with Kawasaki disease?

Coronary artery aneurysm

42. What infectious agent is the cause of a child's low-grade fever, blotchy rash that appears on the cheeks ("slapped-cheek appearance") that may spread to the extremities (sparing the palms and soles) in children?

Parvovirus B19 is the cause of fifth disease or erythema infectiosum.

43. What physical exam findings support the diagnosis of female athlete triad?

(BMI) $<17.5\%$ kg/m^2; bradycardia, orthostatic hypotension, hypothermia, cold extremities, lanugo, parotid gland enlargement or tenderness, epigastric tenderness, eroded tooth enamel, and knuckle or hand calluses (Russell sign)

44. A 12-year-old male presents with a solitary red papule on his arm that has grown rapidly, formed a stalk, and bleeds with light contact. What is the likely diagnosis?

He likely has a pyogenic granuloma. They are benign, acquired, and solitary vascular proliferations that occur most often on the head and neck, the lips and oral cavity, the trunk, and the extremities. They are friable and bleed easily. They start as smooth, red to purple lesions that can be sessile or pedunculated and grow rapidly over several weeks.

45. What is the treatment of choice for uncomplicated lice?

Malathion or permethrin

46. What are the anthropometric findings in growth hormone deficiency (GHD)?

Children with GHD have short stature and drop off in height, then weight, then head circumference on the growth curve with >2.5 SD below mean (corresponds to <0.5 percentile) for height (for chronologic, age, sex, and background) and/or height velocity >2 *SD* below mean (corresponds to approximately <3rd percentile).

47. What potentially allergenic compound is used to make the measles, mumps, and rubella (MMR) immunization?

Gelatin

48. What is the workup when growth hormone deficiency (GHD) is suspected?

TSH for hypothyroidism, electrolytes (low bicarbonate levels may indicate renal tubular acidosis), CBC, ESR, karyotype (in females to rule out Turner syndrome) and radiograph of hand and wrist to determine skeletal age in children (GHD is effectively excluded in children with normal bone age and height velocity.)

49. What diagnosis should be considered if the child has trismus (jaws clamped shut)?

Peritonsillar abscess

50. All children between the ages of 2 and 24 months need further evaluation for their first febrile urinary tract infection with an

Ultrasound to evaluate the kidneys alone. A voiding cystourethrogram (VCUG) to evaluate for vesiculoureteral reflux is NO LONGER recommended for first infection.

51. A few days after eating deli meat at a picnic, a woman who gave birth a few weeks ago develops fever, watery diarrhea, nausea, headache, myalgias, joint aches with a severe headache, and stiff neck. What infection is most concerning for the infant?

Listeria, which has a high mortality rate in neonates, infants, and the elderly. It is extremely common in food supply: *listeria* recovered from 15–70% of raw vegetables, fish, meat, ice cream, and unpasteurized milk. Deli meats are the most common source of infection.

52. What are the most common causes of pneumonia in children between ages 5 and 15 years?

Mycoplasma pneumoniae
Streptococcus pneumoniae
Chlamydia pneumoniae
Viruses are still a major cause.

53. A 17-day-old male presents with decreased feeding; rectal temperature is 100.8° Fahrenheit. Can this child be managed as an outpatient?

No, admission with a septic workup and empiric antibiotics are necessary.

54. Forward-facing child car seats are appropriate for children at what age?

Forward-facing child car seats are appropriate for children aged 2 up to at least age 5, or when they reach the upper weight or height limit of that seat.

55. What is the most common cause of pneumonia in children under age 5?

Viruses. In older infants and up, respiratory syncytial virus is the main viral pathogen.

56. What antibiotics should be used to empirically treat neonatal fever?	Ampicillin and a third generation cephalosporin; the common bacterial causes include Group B Streptococcus, *Escherichia coli*, *Listeria monocytogenes*, *c*oagulase-negative Staphylococcus, and *Treponema pallidum*. *The ampicillin is needed to cover the listeria.*
57. What is the treatment for scabies in children over age 5 years?	5% permethrin cream
58. A newborn has a loud systolic heart murmur heard at the left upper sternal border. What is the likely diagnosis?	This child likely has a patent ductus arteriosus (PDA). If it is persistent PDA after 3 months, it is considered pathologic and should be evaluated for closure.
59. What infection is related to exposure to reptiles?	Pet-associated salmonellosis
60. The appearance of a varicocele on the right side or a varicocele that persists in a supine position is suggestive of	Inferior vena cava (IVC) obstruction due to abdominal or retroperitoneal mass, kidney tumors, IVC or renal vein thrombosis.
61. By what age will flat feet correct spontaneously in children?	One year of age
62. What is the diagnosis when a 7-year-old female develops breast buds and pubic hair?	Precocious puberty; it is defined as the appearance of secondary sexual characteristics before the age of 8 years in girls and 9 years in boys; it is more common in females than males.
63. Fluoride supplementation is recommended for	Preschool children over the age of 6 months. If water not fluorinated, doses include 6 months–3 years: 0.25 mg/day 3 years–6 years: 0.50 mg/day 6 years–18 years 1.0 mg/day

64. What condition is associated with projectile vomiting after eating and poor weight gain in full-term male infants? What color do you expect the vomit to be?

Pyloric stenosis.
Vomit should be nonbilious as the stenosis is located at the pylorus, and above the ampulla of Vater (second part of the duodenum) where bile is released.

65. What is the most common cause of death in ages 1–12 months of life?

Sudden infant death syndrome (SIDS)

66. How should febrile seizures be treated?

Antipyretics

67. "Swimming pool" folliculitis is associated with what organism often found in pools?

Pseudomonas aeruginosa

68. What are the risk factors for SIDS?

Prone and side sleep positions, overheating from heavy clothing and bedding, soft bedding, bed sharing; parental smoking, alcohol, and drug use

69. What noninvasive test should be done in children with acute respiratory distress?

Pulse oximetry

70. What conditions are associated with a "strawberry tongue?"

Kawasaki disease and scarlet fever

71. A 3-year-old African American male has a left flank mass on exam. What is the most concerning etiology?

Wilms tumor (nephroblastoma): most common kidney tumor of childhood; African Americans have a greater risk.

72. Describe the rash in Kawasaki disease.	Erythematous rash that starts at the trunk and spreads to extremities; hands and feet may be swollen and painful.
73. Describe the rash in scarlet fever.	Sandpaper rash, with small papules Rash starts in skin folds, like the neck, axilla, and the groin.
74. How should a young child be positioned to examine the perineum?	Knee-chest position
75. Palpable purpura is a common presenting sign of what illness?	Henoch-Schonlein purpura (HSP); nearly all patients of HSP have palpable purpura.
76. What is the classic tetrad for Henoch Schonlein purpura?	■ Palpable purpura without thrombocytopenia and coagulopathy ■ Arthritis/arthralgia (second most common feature after purpura) ■ Abdominal pain, colicky ■ Renal disease—nephritic syndrome secondary to IgA vasculitis
77. A 12-year-old male is found to have an enlarged liver and brownish rings surrounding his iris. What is the likely diagnosis?	Wilson disease; an autosomal recessive defect in copper excretion resulting in liver deposition and Kayser-Fleischer rings in the eyes
78. Tibial tubercle enlargement and pain with activity in an adolescent is most likely what diagnosis?	Osgood-Schlatter disease
79. In prepubescent females, what is the first line of treatment for labial adhesions?	Topical estrogen

80. An infection with parvovirus B19 in a child with sickle cell anemia can lead to	Aplastic crisis
81. What is the antibiotic of choice for uncomplicated acute otitis media (AOM)?	High dose amoxicillin (80–90 mg/kg/day) *Streptococcus pneumoniae* is the most common bacterial cause of AOM and includes variants with antibiotic resistance.
82. What is the most common infection to cause acute glomerulonephritis in children?	Acute streptococcal throat or skin infection
83. Flesh-colored dome-shaped papules between 2 and 5 mm with central indentation suggest	Molluscum contagiosum, a viral infection in the poxvirus family
84. Which headache type is most common in children?	Migraine
85. What organisms are associated with external otitis?	External otitis, also known as "swimmer's ear, is most often associated with *Pseudomonas aeruginosa* (most common), *Staphylococcus epidermidis*, and *Staphylococcus aureus*.
86. New onset hip pain with a negative x-ray in a child suggests	Transient synovitis, a self-limiting condition that resolves on its own between 1 and 4 weeks. If hip pain persists, then evaluate for Legg–Calve–Perthes disease, as its early stages will not show up on radiograph.
87. What is the antibiotic of choice for complicated AOM?	Augmentin (amoxicillin-clavulanate) Children presenting with AOM with purulent conjunctivitis, children with a history of recurrent AOM, and recent use of β-lactams (higher risk of antibiotic resistance) should receive this.

88. A 3-year-old boy who has had a cold and fever for the last day has a generalized seizure lasting 2 minutes; he is now fine and exam is normal. What is the likely diagnosis?

Febrile seizure; if the patient has pointing neurologic signs, has a repeat seizure within 24 hours, or if the seizure lasts more than 15 minutes, more aggressive work up is needed, including a lumbar puncture (LP).

89. Anaphylaxis including hypotension and respiratory distress due to an insect sting is best treated with what agent?

Systemic epinephrine

90. Where should a pulse be obtained in a child under age 1 year?

Brachial pulse

91. What syndrome is associated with a thin upper lip, a smooth philtrum, flat nasal bridge, growth retardation, clinodactyly (curved digit), and central nervous system (CNS) abnormalities?

Fetal alcohol syndrome

92. Paroxysms of severe coughing with an inspiratory whoop are associated with what preventable infectious disease?

Pertussis ("whooping cough")

93. Regarding the routine screening of asymptomatic adolescents for idiopathic scoliosis, the United States Preventive Services Task Force (USPSTF) and the American Academy of Family Physicians has recommended

Against routine screening

94. Henoch-Schonlein Purpura (HSP) is the most common vasculitis of childhood which rarely causes what organ system to fail?

Renal system failure
HSP is an immunoglobulin A vasculitis that causes nephritic syndrome and can lead to renal failure.

95. A 10-year-old female presents with 2 days of sore throat, fever, and now bilateral knee pain. What is the likely diagnosis?

Acute rheumatic fever (large joint arthritis, carditis, heart valve disease, an erythema marginatum rash, subcutaneous nodules, chorea) is related to a recent group A strep infection.

96. When pertussis is diagnosed, how should close contacts be treated?

Post-exposure prophylaxis (macrolide) and nasopharyngeal specimen regardless of symptoms

97. What malignancies are associated with Down syndrome?

Acute myeloid or lymphoblastic leukemia; Testicular cancer

98. In a patient with egg allergy, which vaccine should be used with caution?

Both inactive and live attenuated influenza vaccine (LAIV) contain trace amounts of egg; they may be used with caution as the amount of egg exposure is considered not significant.

99. A male is born with a hypospadias; is this a contraindication to circumcision?

Yes, contraindications for immediate circumcision include prematurity, genital anomalies, and bleeding disorders.

100. What is the mechanism of action of benzoyl peroxide?

Benzoyl peroxide is an antibacterial drug that acts by releasing free radical oxygen. It is useful in treating inflammatory acne.

101. Indication for the human papilloma virus (HPV) recombinant vaccination includes what population?

Females and males aged 9–26 years

102. Cyclical abdominal cramping in the absence of menstrual blood flow in an adolescent female who is otherwise fully developed suggests what diagnosis?

Imperforate hymen

103. How is the diagnosis of pertussis confirmed?

Polymerase chain reaction (PCR) obtained from a nasopharyngeal swab

104. What is the most common cause of visual impairment in children?

Amblyopia (visual loss due to decreased input, often from strabismus [lazy eye])

105. What class of oral antibiotics should be avoided until after adolescence?

Fluoroquinolones

106. Severe conjunctivitis, keratitis, and visual loss are associated with what infection?

Herpes infections

107. What medication, if administered to a patient with infectious mononucleosis, may cause a maculopapular, petechial, or urticarial rash?

Ampicillin (or amoxicillin)

108. A 4-year-old male presents with a fever (101°F) and sore throat. There is no cough or rhinnorhea. His exam finds tonsillar exudates and painful anterior cervical lymphadenopathy. What is the most likely diagnosis?

Streptococcal pharyngitis

109. An infant presents with excessive tearing and a swelling of the tear duct; what is the likely diagnosis?	Congenital dacryostenosis or congenital naso-lacrimal duct obstruction, which usually self-re-solves by 6 months of age. Treatment consists of milking the lacrimal sac.
110. The development of a "herald patch" on the trunk followed by generalized eruption of salmon-colored lesions in a Christmas tree pattern is associated with what skin condition?	Pityriasis rosea
111. A teenage female shows you a rash on the external surface of her proximal arms that are small papules of keratin with a sandpaper-like feel; what is the likely diagnosis?	Keratosis pilaris; an abrasive ("sandpaper-like," "chicken skin-like," or "goose bump-like") texture of the skin is caused by excess buildup of keratin. Treatment includes lactic acid 12% creams/lotions or topical 40%–50% urea.
112. Screening of vision in young children is designed to identify patients with what condition that causes reduced visual acuity without an identifiable organic lesion of the eye.	Amblyopia; a functional reduction in visual acuity due to abnormal visual development. It has three etiologic classes: strabismus, refractive errors, and deprivational loss from congenital defects (i.e., congenital cataracts, ptosis, congenital corneal opacities, vitreous hemorrhage).
113. What tests can be used to detect strabismus (ocular misalignment) in children under the age of 1 year?	The cover test and the corneal light reflex test
114. Screening for visual disorders (amblyopia, strabismus, and defects in visual acuity) is recommended in children of what age?	Less than 5 years of age

115. Severe sore throat, fever, tonsillar exudates, and posterior chain lymph-adenopathy is associated with what infection?

Infectious mononucleosis

116. Petechiae on the palate of a child or teen is associated with what infections?

Streptococcal pharyngitis and mononucleosis

117. What are the major complications associated with strep throat?

Acute rheumatic fever and post-streptococcocal glomerulonephritis

118. A child who presents with a toxic appearance, muffled voice, fluctuant tonsils, and uvular deviation has what condition?

Peritonsillar abscess

119. Why should children under 1 year of age avoid honey?

Honey may contain *Clostridium botulinum* which, in the immature intestine, can result in neurotoxicity.

120. Acute conjunctivitis is most commonly caused by which virus?

Adenovirus

121. What are the most common causes of bacterial conjunctivitis in children?

Streptococcus pneumoniae, *Haemophilus influenzae*, and *Moraxella catarrhalis*.
Staphylococcus aureus is another cause but is more often seen in adults.

122. Café-au-lait spots are common macular hyper-pigmented lesions in children; if more than 6 are present, what condition should be considered?

Neurofibromatosis type 1

123. What are the cardinal features associated with Marfan syndrome?	Aortic root dilation and ectopic lentis (dislocation of ocular lens)
124. A tall young male presents for a new visit; he has an arm span that exceeds his height, a high-arched palate, pectus excavatum, and hyperextensibility of joints. What condition needs to be investigated?	Marfan syndrome is an inherited connective tissue disorder with unique physical characteristics including an arm span that exceeds height, arachnodactyly ("spider fingers" long thin fingers), ocular lens disorders, a high-arched palate, pectus excavatum, and hyperextensibility of joints.
125. Hypextensibility of joints, stretchy skin, multiple joint dislocations, bruises, and poor wound healing should raise suspicion for	Ehlers-Danlos syndrome
126. What is the treatment of choice for children less than 2 years of age with nasal congestion?	Saline nose drops and rubber suction bulbs; over-the-counter decongestants should not be used.
127. What is the most common cause of fecal incontinence in children?	Functional constipation
128. An infant presents with long delays between bowel movements that are often large and hard; what are the organic causes of constipation in children?	Cystic fibrosis (constipation presents in infancy), Hirschsprung disease (presents in infancy), celiac disease, hypothyroidism. Older children may develop constipation from lead poisoning, developmental delay, abuse, medication side effects.
129. A teen presents with "flashes of light," decreased night vision, and loss of peripheral vision fields. What common inherited condition can cause blindness by age 30?	Retinitis pigmentosa is an inherited condition that causes night blindness due to degeneration of rods resulting in decline of night vision, followed by progressive loss of peripheral fields. It affects 1 in 4,000 people in the United States.

130. In early childhood development, at what age should children know the basic colors and be able to articulate most words?

4 years of age

---

131. At what age should a male with an undescended testicle be referred for urologic evaluation?

Referral should occur if the testicle remains undescended after 6 months, with the plan to repair if it does not descend before 24 months of age.

---

132. A child is found to have an absent testicle; at what age should orchiopexy be performed?

Before 24 months of age

---

133. What test is used to diagnose testicular torsion?

Ultrasound

---

134. In a child with short stature, delayed bone age is found. What conditions should be considered?

A systemic or metabolic disorder (i.e., hypothyroidism)

---

135. What are the signs and symptoms of growth hormone deficiency?

Poor height velocity, slower muscular development, and delayed gross motor milestones (standing, walking, jumping)

---

136. A 2-year-old presents a few days after resolution of an upper respiratory tract infection (URI) with sudden onset of severe intermittent (colicky) abdominal pain characterized by drawing the legs up to the abdomen and crying. What condition should be of concern?

Intussusception

137. At what age do frontal sinuses develop in children?	Frontal sinuses develop around age 10; frontal sinusitis is unusual before age 10.
138. What diagnostic tools are used in the diagnosis of attention deficit hyperactivity disorder?	Vanderbilt Assessment Scale and the Conners Comprehensive Behavior Rating Scales
139. A young child complains of leg pain only during the night; what signs and symptoms are consistent with "growing pains?"	1. The leg pain is bilateral and there is no arthritis. 2. The pain occurs only at night. 3. The child has no limp, pain, or symptoms during the day.
140. What are the common organisms associated with peritonsillar abscess?	Often polymicrobial organisms, including *Streptococcus pyogenes* (group A β-hemolytic Streptococcus), *Streptococcus anginosus*, *Staphylococcus aureus* (including methicillin-resistant Staphylococcus aureus [MRSA]), and anaerobes
141. In addition to inflamed joints, what are the other features of juvenile idiopathic arthritis?	High "quotidian" fevers (pattern of daily fever spikes and spontaneous return to normal temperature), macular salmon pink rash, uveitis
142. A child comes in with > 6 weeks of joint swelling, restricted range of motion, warmth, redness, or pain. What is the likely diagnosis?	Juvenile idiopathic arthritis; lab evaluation will likely show leukocytosis, thrombocytosis, and anemia, elevated ESR or CRP, elevated ferritin.
143. What is the most common cause of diffuse, chronic abdominal pain in a child?	Functional gastrointestinal disorder (FGID); ROME criteria include functional abdominal pain at least 25% of the time and one or more of the following: ■ Some loss of daily functioning ■ Additional somatic symptoms such as headache, limb pain, or difficulty sleeping

144. Under what conditions can a child start using an adult seat belt?

When the seatbelt fits properly, i.e., when the lap belt fits over proximal thighs (not stomach) and upper belt fits across the chest (not the neck)

145. What are the criteria for children to use booster seats?

From age 5 years until the lap and chest seatbelts fit properly

146. A local elementary school has an outbreak of vomiting in the student body. What virus is the likely cause?

Rotavirus, often presenting with vomiting

147. Early sexual activity and childbirth is associated with what outcomes?

Academic deficiencies, lower socioeconomic outcomes, repeat pregnancy, and tendency to single parenthood

148. What are the first objective signs of puberty in girls?

Rapid increase in height, then the development of breast buds

149. What are the first objective signs of puberty in boys?

Testicular enlargement followed by the appearance of pubic hair, enlargement of the penis, and development of sperm

150. An upper GI series shows a "bird's beak" sign in a child. What is the most likely diagnosis?

Midgut volvulus secondary to malrotation around the superior mesenteric artery

151. What are the health risks of bottle feeding at bedtime?

Dental caries

152. Most otitis media is caused by viral infections. What bacteria commonly cause AOM?

Streptococcus pneumoniae, *Haemophilus influenzae*, and *Moraxella catarrhalis*

153.	What are the risks of elevated serum lead levels in children?	Lead toxicity can cause developmental delay, language delay, intellectual disability, behavior issues, hearing loss, and encephalopathy at high levels.
154.	The parent of a bottle-fed infant asks how much formula the baby needs. How many ounces per day does the baby need?	Generally, a term infant needs 2.5 oz/lb/day. Formula contains 20 cal/oz.
155.	Significantly elevated bilirubin levels lead to	Kernicterus
156.	What hip condition affects previously healthy overweight adolescent boys and presents with antalgic gait and resistance to internal rotation of the hips?	Slipped capital femoral epiphyses (SCFE): chronic pain with insidious onset in boys between ages 10 and 16 years. Antalgic gait results from hip pain caused by displaced capital femoral epiphysis from the femoral neck. Pain will occasionally refer to the knees.
157.	What oral medication is used for the treatment of tinea capitis?	Oral griseofulvin or oral terbinafine, as topical treatment of tinea capitis is not effective.
158.	What clinical finding is the most common presenting finding associated with Hodgkin lymphoma?	Painless lymphadenopathy in the neck that feels rubbery and firm
159.	What bacteria is the focus of treatment in adolescent acne?	*Propionibacterium acnes*

160. What condition is associated with a child who has academic performance below IQ, being forgetful or a "daydreamer," and a characteristic 3-Hz generalized spike-and-slow wave pattern on EEG?

Absence seizures

---

161. Idiopathic avascular necrosis of the femoral head in a young child is also known as what condition?

Legg–Calve–Perthes disease

---

162. Where is lymphadenopathy found in infectious mononucleosis?

Posterior cervical chain

---

163. To prevent hemorrhagic disease of the newborn, what medication is given at birth?

Vitamin K, 0.5–1 mg administered intramuscularly

---

164. For mild to moderate croup, what treatment is effective in lowering the risk of progression and intubation?

Dexamethasone

---

165. What is the antidote of choice for iron poisoning?

Deferoxamine

---

166. What clinical manifestations are associated with Down syndrome?

Flattened midface with depressed nasal bridge, slanted palpebral fissures, epicanthic folds, low set ears, single palmar crease, hypotonia, poor Moro reflex, dysplasia of mid phalanx of fifth finger, excessive skin at nape of neck, hyperflexibility of joints, dysplasia of pelvis, Brushfield spots (gray to white spots around the periphery of the iris), intellectual disability, short fingers

167. What macular rash begins on the chest, moves to extremities, and converts to crops of vesicles on erythematous bases ("dewdrops on a rose petal")?

Varicella (chickenpox)

168. What illness begins initially with a macular rash that becomes vesicular and occurs on the palms of the hands and plantar aspects of the feet?

Hand-foot-and-mouth disease caused by coxsackievirus. The illness typically has a 1-day prodrome of fever, anorexia, malaise, abdominal pain, and upper respiratory symptoms.

169. What infection may induce fetal hydrops in a pregnant woman?

Erythema infectiosum

170. An infant presents with an erythematous diaper rash that involves the skin folds and has "satellite lesions" is most likely caused by what organism?

Candida albicans

171. A diaper rash that is erythematous and prominent on the convex surfaces but spares the skin folds is most likely what kind of rash?

Irritant dermatitis

172. What do clinical manifestations of Kawasaki disease include?

High fevers minimally responsive to antipyretics and unexplained source lasting 5 days or more, nonexudative conjunctivitis, lip cracking and fissuring, strawberry tongue, cervical lymphadenopathy, arthralgias, exanthema, redness and swelling of the hands and feet, can include palms and soles

173. In a child with Kawasaki disease, what organ system complication is most worrisome?

Coronary artery aneurysm is the main complication. However, myocarditis, pericarditis, valvular heart disease, and coronary arteritis, acute MI, arrhythmia, and death can also occur. Coronary artery thrombosis is the leading cause of death in Kawasaki disease (and why aspirin is prescribed).

174. With premature infants, what modifications need to be made to the immunization schedule?

Standard immunization schedule should continue just like a full-term well baby. The only exception is the Hepatitis B vaccine, which should be delayed by 1 month.

175. A child is seen in the Emergency Department with a spiral fracture and multiple injuries in different stages of healing. What diagnosis should be considered?

Child abuse

176. Coarctation of the aorta will be suggested by what finding on chest x-ray?

Rib notching on a chest radiograph is suggestive of coarctation of the aorta.

177. What are the common complications of cystic fibrosis?

Meconium ileus present at birth, chronic cough and wheezing with copious mucus production, pancreatic insufficiency, insulin-dependent diabetes mellitus, retarded growth, and infertility

178. In a child with concerning clinical features, what test is used to diagnose cystic fibrosis?

Sweat chloride test

179. A young adult with a cough who develops pleuritic chest pain, but without rales on exam is suspicious for *Mycoplasma* infection. What antibiotic should be used first line?

A macrolide antibiotic

180. Why does the AAFP and the AAP recommend withholding whole milk to infants younger than 1 year of age?

It may induce iron deficiency anemia.

181. A 5-year-old keeps waking at night complaining of rectal itching; you suspect pinworms (*Enterobius vermicularis*). What are the treatment options for pinworms?

Albendazole, mebendazole, or pyrantel pamoate (over the counter)

182. What condition in a child under 4 years of age is associated with farm animal contact or eating undercooked chicken, resulting in bloody diarrhea?

Campylobacter infection

183. An infant has a "C shaped" foot, with medial deviation (adduction) of the distal foot while the hindfoot remains in a normal position forming a concavity of the medial aspect of the foot. What is the likely diagnosis?

Metatarsus adductus is the most common congential foot abnormality in children.

184. An unvaccinated child presents with some respiratory distress and an unusual inspiratory "whoop." What is the likely diagnosis and treatment?

This child likely has whooping cough caused by a *Bordetella pertussis* infection, which is treated with a macrolide antibiotic.

185. What is the drug of choice for the treatment of impetigo with a small number of lesions?

Topical mupirocin

186. The parents of an infant with an umbilical hernia are concerned and want him to have surgery. What should you tell them about the natural course of umbilical hernias in children?

Umbilical hernias found in infancy most often resolve by 1 year of age.

187. A delay in growth and development that patterns after parental growth and development suggests what condition?

Genetic short stature

188. In children, what is the most common malignancy?

Acute lymphoblastic leukemia (ALL)

189. When should iron-fortified cereals be the first solid food introduced to young infants?

Between 4 and 6 months of age

190. In a very premature infant, what is the danger of excessive oxygen administration?

Retinopathy of prematurity (ROP)

191. For children with cradle cap, what is the treatment of choice?

1% hydrocortisone cream

192. What congenital feature found in young boys increases the risk of recurrent urinary tract infections?

Posterior urethral valves

193. A 16-year-old boy presents with a rash on his back that follows a "Christmas tree" pattern that began as a pink macular spot. What is the likely condition?

Pityriasis rosea

194. What is the next course of treatment for a 9-year-old female with asthma who has 4 days of wheezing despite using her rescue inhaler every 4 to 6 hours with only temporary improvement?

Oral steroids

195. Lower leg pain in an athlete that resolves with rest with tenderness over the middle to distal third of the tibia is consistent with what?

Medial tibial stress syndrome (shin splints)

196. Lower leg pain in an athlete that gets worse with exercise who cannot hop 10 times on the affected leg due to pain needs testing for what condition?

Stress fracture; x-ray may not turn positive until >2 weeks of pain.

197. In January, you see a 5-month-old male with fever, cough, runny nose, and wheezing. What is the likely infection?

Bronchiolitis caused by respiratory syncytial virus (RSV)

198. A 2-year-old male presents with a barky cough and stridor with slight retractions; his cough was preceded by 2 days of mild cold symptoms. What is the likely diagnosis?

Croup, caused by parainfluenza virus; treatment includes dexamethasone and if concerned, epinephrine.

199. What organism causes hand-foot-and-mouth disease?

Coxsackievirus A16

200. By what age should the anterior fontanel close?

12 months of age

201. A 5-year-old internationally adopted male presents with drooling and difficulty breathing; lateral neck x-ray shows a "positive thumb sign." What is the likely diagnosis?

Epiglottitis

202. A 13-year-old male presents with unilateral breast tenderness; the remainder of his exam is normal. What is the likely diagnosis?

Benign gynecomastia of adolescence; treatment involves reassurance, and encouragement to not repeatedly irritate the breast.

203. A 3-year-old male presents with a unilateral purulent, malodorous, and bloody nasal discharge. What is the likely cause?

A foreign body

204. On the 12-month visit, you notice a child has femoral anteversion ("toeing-in"). What treatment should be initiated?

Observation; most cases resolve by age 8 years.

205. Parents report their child wakes at night screaming, with eyes open, but seems unable to see and appears scared and confused. What is the likely diagnosis?

Night terrors are associated with these symptoms and are related to a child not getting enough sleep or having fever. It occurs in Stage 3 and 4 of nonrapid eye movement (NREM) sleep.

206. An under-immunized child presents with URI symptoms including a cough, bilateral conjunctivitis, and runny nose. His exam is significant for an erythematous rash that begins at the neck, and small white spots on an erythematous base on the buccal mucosa. What is the likely diagnosis?

Measles. The oral findings are Koplik spots, pathognamonic signs of measles (rubeola).
Other symptoms of measles include the three Cs (cough, coryza, conjunctivitis), high fever, and a maculopapular rash.

207. What is a chronic pruritic superficial inflammation of the skin with a relapsing and remitting pattern, also affecting the antecubital and popliteal fossa called?

Atopic dermatitis

208. "Currant jelly" stool is suggestive what diagnosis?

Intussusception

209. A child that "walks" his hands and arms forward to assist in rising from a sitting position is associated with what condition?

Duchenne muscular dystrophy
This pattern of movement is the Gower sign, and occurs due to diminished hip and thigh muscle strength from the disease.

210. What is the mechanism of injury associated with "nursemaid's elbow?"

Subluxation of the radial head past the annular ligament when a child's fully extended arm is pulled in an upward direction. The annular ligament becomes trapped in the radiohumeral joint.

211. What is the most common malignant pediatric bone tumor?

Osteosarcoma

212. Chronic unilateral limb pain that awakens a child from sleep suggests what diagnosis?

Osteosarcoma

213. Patellofemoral syndrome most commonly presents with what clinical signs?

Chronic diffuse anterior knee pain that worsens with squatting, running (especially downhill), stairs, and getting up from a chair after sitting for some time

214. Patellofemoral syndrome responds to rehabilitation of what muscle group?

Quadricep muscles

215. Isotretinoin requires monitoring of what blood tests?

Pregnancy (is a teratogen), LFTs, lipids

216. The most common cause of occult bacteremia in children?

Streptococcus pneumoniae

217. How does a child with occult bacteremia present?	Relatively well-appearing young child (usually < 3 years) with high fevers (≥ 39°C) and unknown source.
218. What vaccination should not be given at the same time as varicella as it may decrease the effectiveness of the varicella vaccine?	MMR vaccine
219. What are the most common organisms associated with periorbital cellulitis in vaccinated children?	*Staphylococcus aureus, Streptococcus pneumoniae*
220. What diagnosis presents with a lack of attachment to others, preoccupation with inanimate objects, avoidance of eye contact, resistance to change, outburst of temper, repetitive often self-destructive acts, and delayed speech development?	Autism
221. On routine newborn exam, a painless cystic structure is found in the scrotum that transilluminates. What is the likely diagnosis?	Hydrocele, a collection of peritoneal fluid between the parietal and visceral layers of the tunica vaginalis; Most hydroceles seen in newborns resolve during the first year of life.
222. What is the most common pediatric immunodeficiency?	IgA deficiency
223. Head lice is passed on by what mode of transmission?	Person-to-person contact

224. What is the drug of choice for treating dog bites?

Amoxicillin-clavulanate (Augmentin)

225. What percentage of females are believed to be sexually assaulted or abused by age 18?

12%–25%

226. A 1-month-old infant presents with cyclic paroxysms of crying, abdominal pain, and irritability that is difficult to console and resolves on its own by age 4 months. What is the likely diagnosis?

Infant colic

227. Pediatric fluid resuscitation for an emergent situation should be treated with what fluid and bolused at what rate?

20 mL/kg of lactated Ringer solution or 0.9% sodium chloride solution rapidly infused intravenously

228. Amblyopia is a reduction in visual acuity because of abnormal visual development in the absence of a structural or pathologic abnormality of the eye, not correctable by eyeglasses or contact lenses. How is this treated?

Glasses and patching
A patch is placed over the normal preferred eye, forcing the use of the suppressed eye.

229. How is pseudostrabismus diagnosed?

Symmetric corneal light reflex

230. Who should be screened for sexually transmitted infections (STIs)?	Sexually transmitted diseases including gonorrhea and chlamydia should be screened for in sexually active women age 24 years and younger and in older women who are at increased risk for infection; for men, evidence is lacking, but screening is encouraged.
231. What are the discharge criteria for a premature infant from the neonatal unit?	1. Body temperature is maintained. 2. Weight gain of 10–30 g/day is achieved. 3. No medications require hospital management. 4. No major changes in medications or oxygen administration have occurred. 5. No recent episodes of apnea or bradycardia have occurred.
232. Impetigo is caused by what organisms?	*Staphylococcus aureus* is the primary pathogen. Group A β-*hemolytic Streptococcus* is less common but can also cause impetigo, at times, in combination with *S. aureus*.
233. In young athletes, what is the most common cause of sudden cardiac death?	Hypertrophic cardiomyopathy
234. What type of murmur should suggest hypertrophic cardiomyopathy?	A systolic ejection murmur at the left upper sternal border that increases in intensity with a Valsalva maneuver
235. An erythematous wheal with a central papule that comes and goes in newborns is called	*Erythema toxicum*
236. What is the thin yellow fluid that presents in the mother's breast before and for a few days after birth called?	Colostrum

237. What components in colostrum are important to a baby's health?

Colostrum is a high-calorie and high-protein substance containing maternal antibodies.

238. What are the five criteria used when calculating an Apgar score?

Color, heart rate, respiration, reflex response, and muscle tone

239. With a pertussis infection, what are the three stages and their implications?

Catarrhal stage: Sneezing, lacrimation, coryza, hacking cough especially at night, fever is rare. Lasts 1 to 2 weeks. Antibiotics may shorten illness and infectious state.

Paroxysmal stage: Cough increases in severity, 5–15 consecutive coughs occur in a single expiration followed by a "whoop"—a hurried deep inspiration—and copious amounts of mucus may be expelled. Can last between 2 and 8 weeks. Antibiotics provide no benefit to the patient.

Convalescent stage: Cough starts to improve, paroxysms not as frequent or severe, patient looks and feels better. Lasts from a few weeks to months.

240. What condition may occur from aspirin use in children with respiratory infections?

Reye syndrome

241. What is the most common type of child abuse?

Neglect is most common (~75% of abuse) and includes physical neglect (not providing basic necessities such as food and clothes), medical neglect (not meeting basic medical needs), emotional neglect (lack of support, security, encouragement), and educational/developmental neglect (not providing experiences to promote education).

242. What is a common cause of unilateral heel pain in a 13-year-old male that has come on gradually over the last few weeks, and hurts now with activity and with rest?

Sever syndrome: an inflammation of the calcaneal growth plate, typically occurring in teens who are active. Symptoms resolve on their own when the activity is lessened or the growth plate closes.

243. A 4-year-old presents with 2 months of arthralgias, fever, fatigue, malaise, myalgias, weight loss, morning stiffness, and rash. What condition needs to be ruled out?

Juvenile rheumatoid arthritis

244. What is the initial treatment for Kawasaki disease?

IVIG and aspirin

245. What is the most common gastrointestinal (GI) complication associated with Henoch Scholein purpura?

Intussusception

246. What factor increases the risk for AOM?

Age is the greatest risk factor. AOM peaks between 6 and 18 months and declines in school-age children and adolescents. Other factors include
- Attendance at day care centers
- Lack of or limited breastfeeding
- Exposure to cigarette use
- Race and ethnicity—Native American, Alaskan/Canadian Eskimo descent, indigenous Australian children

247. What test should you perform in office for a child with proteinuria?

A negative dip stick on first morning voided specimen can rule out pathologic causes of pediatric proteinuria.

CHAPTER 2 Internal Medicine

1. What condition presents with hypertension, hypernatremia, and hypokalemia?

Hyperaldosteronism from adrenal tumors (Cushing disease) will cause sodium retention and potassium excretion.

2. According to the United States Preventive Services Task Force (USPSTF), what is the breast cancer screening recommendation for women?

Biennial (every other year) between age 50 and 74 years

3. Foot pain with tenderness of the medial calcaneus that is worse when first getting out of bed or after sitting for a long rest without history of trauma is likely what condition?

Plantar fasciitis

4. What conditions are commonly associated with a normal-MCV anemia?

Anemia of chronic disease, chronic renal disease, hypothyroidism

5. What special steps must be completed for diabetics requiring insulin to obtain a commercial drivers license?

Diabetics requiring insulin must apply for and receive an exemption from the Federal Motor Carrier Safety Administration (FMCSA).

6. What are the common presenting symptoms of dengue fever?

Dengue fever presents 3 to 7 days after exposure with high fever (>38.5°C—may be biphasic), headache, cough, sore throat/nasal congestion, relative bradycardia (typically seen in the febrile phase), abdominal pain, and vomiting, myalgia/arthralgia, lethargy, joint pain, and rash

7. What visual fields are affected by macular degeneration?

Macular degeneration causes loss of *central* vision.

8. A young woman returns from a recent trip to Brazil with diffuse arthralgias and conjunctivitis. What condition would cause worry if she were pregnant?

Zika virus infection; its symptoms include fever, myalgia, joint pain, conjunctivitis, retroocular pain, and maculopapular rash.

9. Aspartate transaminase (AST) and alanine transaminase (ALT) findings consistent with chronic alcohol abuse show what ratio?

An AST-to-ALT ratio > 2.0

10. What are the drugs of choice for an acute asthma exacerbation?

Inhaled β-agonists and systemic corticosteroids are indicated for mild, moderate, and severe asthma exacerbations.

11. According to the USPSTF, what are the current testicular cancer screening recommendations?

Recommends against screening for testicular cancer in adolescent or adult men

12. Which patients with joint replacements need antibiotic use before a dental procedure?

None. The American Dental Association recommend not routinely using antibiotics for SBE prophylaxis or prosthetic joint replacement unless the joint replacement was highly complicated and with the advice of the orthopedic surgeon.

13. What is Addison disease due to?

Adrenal insufficiency (AI) is associated with fatigue, abdominal pain, depression, cold intolerance, hyponatremia, and hyperkalemia, which are a result of low serum cortisol and high adrenocorticotropic hormone (ACTH).

14. Which cardiac conditions support the use of antibiotics before dental procedures?

Indications for antibiotics needed before a dental procedure include prosthetic cardiac valve or prosthetic material used for cardiac valve repair, a history of infective endocarditis, a cardiac transplant that develops cardiac valvulopathy, congenital heart disease, unrepaired cyanotic congenital heart disease, including palliative shunts and conduits, a completely repaired congenital heart defect with prosthetic material or device, whether placed by surgery or by catheter intervention during the first six months after the procedure, any repaired congenital heart defect with residual defect or a prosthetic device.

15. How does Meckel diverticulum most commonly present?

Meckel diverticulum is the most common congenital gastrointestinal (GI) tract anomaly. It is typically a blind segment of bowel occurring in the distal ileum. It most commonly presents as painless rectal bleeding and can be associated with vomiting from intussusception or volvulus, and/or fever, similar to the presentation of an appendicitis.

16. According to the USPSTF, what are the colorectal cancer screening recommendations?

Screening for colorectal cancer using fecal occult blood testing, sigmoidoscopy, or colonoscopy in adults, beginning at age 50 years and continuing until age 75 years

17. A patient presents with erythema migrans and a flulike illness. He is found to have retinal hemorrhages. What is the likely cause?

Babesiosis presents with a gradual onset of malaise and fatigue, fever up to 105°F (40.6°C) after recent tick bite transfusion. Common symptoms include chills, sweats, headache, anorexia, nonproductive cough, arthralgia, and nausea. Less common symptoms include vomiting, sore throat, abdominal pain, conjunctival injection, photophobia, weight loss, emotional lability, depression, and hyperesthesia. Jaundice and retinopathy with splinter hemorrhages and retinal infarcts can occur.

18. Waldenström macroglobulinemia is similar to multiple myeloma with what difference?

Waldenström macroglobulinemia presents like multiple myeloma, but there are no bony lytic lesions as in multiple myeloma.

19. What condition can present in a young woman who has just moved to the United States from Japan with a diffuse vasculitis and oral ulcers?

Behcet syndrome; presents with exacerbations and remissions of symptoms; often, the disease is silent between flares. It can affect all types of vessels, and various parts of the body. It can cause oral and genital mucocutaneous ulcerations, skin rashes, arthritis, thrombophlebitis, uveitis, colitis, and neurologic symptoms. It is rare in the United States, but common in Japan and the Middle East.

20. What test of bone metabolism is commonly normal when concerned about multiple myeloma and bone lesions?

Alkaline phosphatase is often normal even with bone lesions. Symptoms and signs of multiple myeloma include bone pain, anemia, elevated creatinine, Bence Jones proteinuria, and an M-band spike on serum protein electrophoresis (SPEP).

21. A patient with a diastolic murmur is found to have a bicuspid aortic valve (BAV). What are the risks of this genetic anomaly?

A BAV is an abnormal formation of the aortic valve that contains two valve leaflets instead of the usual three; it increases the risk of aortic aneurysms, aortic stenosis, and aortic insufficiency.

22. In atrial fibrillation, what are the $CHADS_2$ criteria for prevention of stroke?

$CHADS_2$ criteria for stroke risk:
Congestive heart failure (1 point)
Hypertension (1 point)
Age ≥ 75 (1 point)
Diabetes (1 point)
Prior stroke/transient ischemic attack (TIA) (2 points)

23. A 68-year-old smoker presents with painless hematuria. What diagnosis must be ruled out by cystoscopy?

Bladder cancer, most commonly transitional cell carcinoma, is the most worrisome cause of painless hematuria in a smoker.

24. In CHADS$_2$, what score recommends initiation of anticoagulation to prevent stroke in atrial fibrillation?

CHADS$_2$ criteria for stroke risk:
Congestive heart failure (1 point)
Hypertension (1 point)
Age $\geq$ 75 (1 point)
Diabetes (1 point)
Prior stroke/TIA (2 points)

Score	Risk of stroke per year %
0	1.9
1	2.8
2	4.0
3	5.9
4	8.5
5	12.5
6	18.2

Recommended therapy includes:

Score	Anticoagulation therapy
0	Aspirin
1–2	Aspirin or anticoagulant
3 +	Anticoagulant

The main criticism of the CHADS$_2$ criteria is that an individual with atrial fibrillation and a previous history of stroke, but no other risk factors (i.e., CHADS$_2$ score 2), is only classified as moderate risk, whereas that person is in fact at high risk for another stroke.

25. Heel pain over the lateral calcaneus that worsens with activity is consistent with what diagnosis?

Calcaneal stress fracture

26. According to USPSTF, what are the current lung cancer screening recommendations?

Annual screening for lung cancer with low-dose computed tomography in adults aged 55–80 years who have a 30 pack-year smoking history and currently smoke or who have quit within the past 15 years. Screening should be discontinued once a person has not smoked for 15 years or develops a health problem that substantially limits life expectancy or the ability or willingness to have curative lung surgery.

27. What is the finding on a complete blood count that implies a vitamin B_{12} or folate deficiency?

Macrocytosis (mean cell volume [MCV] > 100 fL)

28. Ankle pain posterior to the medial malleolus that radiates to the arch and heel and is associated with tightness, burning, tingling, and numbness that worsens during standing or activity is likely what condition?

Tarsal tunnel syndrome; diagnosis can be confirmed with a compression test of applying pressure to the tarsal tunnel for 60 seconds to reproduce symptoms.

29. Early vitamin B_{12} deficiency may be associated with the elevation of what two compounds?

Elevation of methylmalonic acid and homocysteine may be a precursor to vitamin B_{12} deficiency.

30. What test should be done to discern if shoulder pain is due to a cervical radiculopathy?

Spurling test: laterally flex the patient's neck 30 degrees to the affected side and then apply a downward axial compression taking care not to laterally flex the neck any further; reproduction of symptoms rules in cervical radiculopathy.

31. What finding noted on lumbar puncture samples is indicative of subarachnoid hemorrhage?

Xanthochromia noted on lumbar puncture indicates subarachnoid hemorrhage (cerebral spinal fluid does *not* clear from tube 1 to tube 4—as is seen in traumatic taps).

32. Hepatic vein obstruction causing right upper quadrant (RUQ) abdominal pain, portal hypertension, hepatomegaly, and ascites is called what?

Budd-Chiari syndrome; it is seen in patients with inherited thrombophilia or hypercoagulable states, malignancy, and pregnancy.

33. At what time should antiviral medication be initiated in HIV patients?

AIDS antiviral therapy should be initiated on all patients at the time of diagnosis regardless of their CD4 counts.

34. Episodes of overeating with loss of control, followed by compensatory behaviors such as self-induced vomiting and misuse of laxatives is called what?

Bulimia nervosa; risk factors include female gender, body dissatisfaction, severe life stressors, low self-esteem, pressure to be thin, perfectionist or obsessive thinking, poor impulse control, substance abuse, family history of substance abuse, affective disorders; sexual abuse is not causally related to bulimia.

35. What findings are associated with adrenal hyperplasia?

Adrenal hyperplasia causes inadequate aldosterone and cortisone production, leading to low sodium levels and elevated potassium levels.

36. What is diffuse interstitial lung disease (DILD)?

DILD is a diverse group of chronic progressive lung diseases associated with alveolar inflammation and/or potentially irreversible pulmonary fibrosis. Causes include environmental, occupational, or drug-associated disease and some systemic disorders (e.g., sarcoidosis, Wegener granulomatosis, collagen vascular disease)

37. What is the drug of choice for torsades de pointes?

Magnesium sulfate, to increase heart rate, which will shorten the QT interval. A lengthened QT interval is the common etiology of torsades de pointes.

38. A 26-year-old male patient has postprandial abdominal pain that is not improved by proton pump inhibitors; there is no weight loss or other findings. What is the likely diagnosis?

Functional dyspepsia: bothersome postprandial fullness, early satiety, or epigastric pain/burning in the absence of causative structural disease (to include normal upper endoscopy) for the preceding 3 months with initial symptom onset at least 6 months prior to diagnosis

39. What are the common side effects of metformin?

Common side effects include GI disturbances and B_{12} deficiency. Rarely, lactic acidosis may occur.

40. A patient has numerous clinically atypical nevi covering his chest, abdomen, and back and is diagnosed with atypical nevus syndrome. What disease risk is increased by having this syndrome?

Malignant melanoma

41. What treatment should be given with a needlestick injury when the source is hepatitis B positive?

HBIG (hepatitis immune globulin), if the person stuck has negative hepatitis B titers. Give hepatitis B vaccine in three series if not previously immunized and HIV prophylaxis if patient status is unknown.

42. According to the USPSTF, what are the current osteoporosis screening recommendations?

Screening for osteoporosis in women aged 65 years and older and in younger women whose fracture risk is equal to or greater than that of a 65-year-old white woman who has no additional risk factors

43. Following a head injury, a patient has polyuria and increased thirst. What condition can induce a decreased secretion of antidiuretic hormone (vasopressin) production?

Diabetes insipidus (DI) is a condition in which there is reduced ability to concentrate the urine due to impaired reabsorption of water in the renal collecting tubules. Symptoms include polyuria and increased thirst. Two main forms of DI include central DI (CDI), which is due to vasopressin (antidiuretic hormone or ADH) deficiency seen following head trauma or related to tumor and nephrogenic DI (NDI), which represents renal tubule unresponsiveness to vasopressin/ADH. DI can be induced by pregnancy, known as gestational DI (GDI).

44. When determining preoperative risk, what exercise tolerance is considered adequate?

Preoperative evaluation is usually sufficient if patient is capable of $\geq$ 4 METS (the ability to climb 4 flights of stairs or walk 4 miles/hr).

Chapter **2** Internal Medicine | **45**

45. What are the different types of hyperparathyroidism (HPT)?

Primary HPT: intrinsic parathyroid gland dysfunction resulting in excessive secretions of parathyroid hormone (PTH).

Secondary HPT is due to vitamin D deficiency or renal failure inducing hypocalcemia resulting in excessive secretion of PTH.

Tertiary HPT is due to longstanding secondary HPT resulting in hyperfunction of the parathyroid gland.

46. What conditions and laboratory findings are associated with celiac disease?

Type 1 diabetics, thyroid disease, and rheumatoid arthritis

Dermatitis herpetiformis

Unexplained anemia

Detected with antiendomysial antibodies (IgA antiendomysial antibodies [IgA anti-EmA]) and IgA anti–tissue transglutaminase (IgA anti-TTG)

Diagnosis should be confirmed with biopsy of the distal duodenum, which will show villous flattening.

47. What tests should be ordered when hypercalcemia is found incidentally?

PTH, creatinine, 25OH vitamin D level

48. What blood indices are seen in iron deficiency anemia?

Microcytic, hypochromic indices

Decreased ferritin levels

Elevated total iron-binding capacity (TIBC)

Low iron levels

49. A patient is found to have hypercalcemia and an elevated parathyroid hormone; what is the likely diagnosis?

Primary hyperparathyroidism (HPT); ultrasound of the thyroid and parathyroid glands should be obtained next.

50. What class of medication is used in the treatment of Paget disease?

Antiresorptive agents such as bisphosphonates and calcitonin are used in Paget disease of the bone.

51. A 58-year-old male has drug-resistant hypertension (BP 160/100 on triple antihypertensive therapy) and hypokalemia. What condition is a common cause of resistant hypertension with hypokalemia?

Conn syndrome (primary aldosteronism) is due to excess aldosterone production by the adrenal glands, resulting in hypokalemia and drug-resistant hypertension. Workup includes determination of the aldosterone to renin ratio (ARR), metabolic panel (for sodium, potassium, bicarbonate, and creatinine), plasma renin activity (PRA), plasma aldosterone concentration (PAC). ARR > 30 requires further workup, including CT of the adrenals.

52. What serious neurologic side effect is associated with Tramadol?

Seizures

53. What is the etiology of Addison disease?

Addison disease is a primary adrenal gland insufficiency due to destruction of the adrenal cells with inadequate secretion of glucocorticoids and mineralocorticoids, most often due to autoimmune-induced gland destruction.

54. In adults over age 65 years, what is the most common cause of blindness?

Age-related macular degeneration

55. What is the likely diagnosis in a patient with hyponatremia, hyperkalemia, and hyperpigmentation of the skin on areas with recurrent pressure and trauma?

Addison disease; patients develop hyperpigmentation in high-friction areas (extensor surfaces, plantar or palmar creases, dental-gingival margins, buccal and vaginal mucosae, lips, areolae, pressure points, scars; women may lose hair) along with adrenocortical insufficiency resulting in hyponatremia and hyperkalemia.

56. What are common risk factors for osteoporosis?

Female sex
Advanced age
Late menarche
Early menopause
Cigarette smoking
Family history of premature fractures
Low body mass index (BMI)
Corticosteroid use
Caucasian and Asian ethnicity
Heavy ethanol use

57. A few days after a recent upper respiratory infection (URI), a patient presents with a rash that begins on the back of hands and top of the feet and within 24 hours spreads centrally. The lesions, sharply demarcated and pink, turn from macules to papules, then plaques and increase in number rapidly. What is the likely diagnosis?

Erythema multiforme: this rash is seen following a viral infection (often herpes simplex), is sharply demarcated, round, red/pink, and flat (macules), and starts on the back of the hands and tops of the feet. The rash quickly spreads centrally, and becomes papules and ultimately forms plaques that increase in diameter. These lesions evolve within 72 hours. Mucous membranes may be involved.

58. According to the USPSTF, what are the current prostate cancer recommendations?

The USPSTF recommends that clinicians inform men ages 55 to 69 years about the potential benefits and harms of prostate-specific antigen (PSA)–based screening for prostate cancer.

59. What is the antibiotic of choice for treatment of outpatient dental infections?

Amoxicillin: 500 mg TID for 7–10 days; in children, 40–60 mg/kg/day divided TID
If penicillin-allergic, use clindamycin 300 mg PO TID for 7 days.

60. A patient has a rash on the hip that is round plaque with central clearing; it started small and seems to be expanding. There is no pain or itch. What is the likely diagnosis?

Erythema annulare centrifugum (EAC) is an annular or figurate erythematous plaque with central clearing and a characteristic trailing scale along the inner border; it is often present on the trunk, upper arms, hips, or lower extremities and is thought to be a hypersensitivity reaction. Common associations include some medications (NSAIDs), tinea pedis, and onychomycosis. It is rarely associated with malignancy.

61. What class of analgesic medication can induce acute renal insufficiency?

Nonsteroidal antiinflammatory agents can induce an elevation in creatinine and induce renal insufficiency, especially in the elderly.

62. A 26-year-old female presents with bilateral, erythematous, tender nodules on her lower legs that evolve in color similar to bruises. What is the likely cause?

Erythema nodosum is a delayed-type hypersensitivity reaction or an autoimmune reaction that may evolve into a panniculitis that affects subcutaneous fat.

63. What class of antihypertensive medications can induce renal failure in patients with renovascular hypertension?

Angiotensin converting enzyme (ACE) inhibitors (enalapril, lisinopril, moexipril, trandolapril)

64. What common medications are associated with erythema nodosum?

Oral contraceptives and amoxicillin

65. B-type natriuretic peptide is used to differentiate what conditions that present with shortness of breath?

Congestive heart failure (>400 pg/mL) versus chronic obstructive pulmonary disease (COPD) (<100 pg/mL)

66. What causes unilateral ear fullness, giving a clogged or "underwater" sensation and muffled sounds from that ear and can last for weeks?

Eustachian tube dysfunction

67. What condition in women is associated with urinary frequency, urgency, dysuria, dyspareunia, and a negative urine culture?

Interstitial cystitis

68. What are the common physical and clinical signs of Cushing syndrome?

Physical signs include moon face, weight gain, "buffalo" hump, menstrual irregularities, hirsutism, striae, and acne; laboratory findings include hypernatremia and hypokalemia.

69. What are the clinical and laboratory criteria for diagnosis of interstitial cystitis?

The absence of genital infections or neoplastic disease
No history of radiation, tuberculosis, or chemical cystitis
Testing includes anesthetic bladder challenge and cystoscopy.
Antibiotics should not be used.

70. What is the most common cause of Cushing syndrome?

Exogenous corticosteroid use in the form of steroids

71. When should asymptomatic bacteriuria (significant bacteriuria not accompanied by signs and symptoms referable to urinary tract infection) be treated with antibiotics?

Treat asymptomatic bacteriuria with antibiotics only in pregnancy, in renal transplant patients, and before urologic procedures.

72. When prescribing iron supplementation, what states can alter absorption?	Acidic environment Absorption is increased in an acid environment (often given with ascorbic acid [vitamin C]) and decreased by antacids, soy protein, calcium, tannin (tea), and phytates (in bran).
73. What is fibromyalgia?	Chronic, widespread noninflammatory musculoskeletal pain syndrome believed to be a disorder of altered central pain regulation
74. What are the drugs of choice to treat *Mycoplasma pneumonia*?	Mycoplasma is susceptible to macrolide antibiotics (i.e., azithromycin) and some tetracyclines (i.e., doxycycline).
75. What is the drug of choice for polycystic ovary syndrome (PCOS)?	Metformin; it helps preserve fertility and reduces insulin levels.
76. What are the evidence-based treatments for fibromyalgia?	Cognitive behavioral therapy, aerobic exercise, and sleep hygiene
77. Rhinitis medicamentosa (rebound congestion) is secondary with the use of	Chronic (>3 days) intranasal decongestants such as phenylephrine
78. In the empiric treatment of gastroesophageal reflux disease (GERD), how long should a proton pump inhibitor (PPI) be used before weaning off?	8 weeks
79. How many days after exposure to genital herpes is its incubation period?	4 days
80. What are the uncommon adverse effects of long-term PPI use?	Hypomagnesemia, B12 deficiency, increased rates of pneumonia, *Clostridium difficile* infection, osteoporosis

81. To help decrease the risk of postherpetic neuralgia, within what time frame should antiviral therapy be started?

3 days (72 hours)

82. What are the most important lifestyle changes for the treatment of GERD?

Weight loss, elimination of trigger foods, smoking cessation, elevation of the head of the bed, not reclining within 2 hours of eating, stress reduction.

83. Indications for bariatric surgery include

BMI > 35 and medical comorbidities (diabetes, hypertension, obstructive sleep apnea, etc.)
BMI > 40 or 100% over ideal weight without associated medical problems
Alcohol abuse is a contraindication to surgery.

84. What are the risk factors for Barrett esophagitis?

Age > 50, male, symptoms over 5 years, and obesity

85. What is the vector for human ehrlichiosis?

Lone star ticks

86. Is diagnosing and treating *Helicobacter pylori* infection beneficial in GERD treatment?

Treating *H. pylori* may make GERD symptoms worse; testing and treatment is not recommended (the majority of US citizens are colonized with *H. pylori*, which may be protective against GERD)

87. What is the vector for schistosomiasis?

Freshwater snails
It is an infection of flatworm (trematodes) and occurs in Africa, Asia, and South America.

88. What are the three causes of peptic ulcer disease?

H. pylori infection, chronic NSAID use (including low-dose aspirin), and hypersecretion syndromes; alcohol, tobacco, and stress are risk factors, but are not by themselves considered causative.

89. What is the vector for transmission of the Yersinia pestis (plague)?

Fleas
Transmission occurs mostly in the Southwestern United States and Peru.

90. What is the risk low-dose, enteric-coated aspirin will induce a peptic ulcer?

It is estimated that chronic low-dose aspirin will induce a peptic ulcer in 3 out of 1,000 patients.

91. What is the common cause of a gnawing abdominal pain after eating?

Peptic ulcer disease; symptoms that should require further investigation before treatment include episodic gnawing or burning epigastric pain, pain occurring after meals or on empty stomach, and nocturnal pain.

92. What is the drug of choice for patients with end-stage (FEV$_1$ < 1.0 L or less and a Pao$_2$ of 60 mm Hg or less) that improves mortality?

Oxygen
β-agonists can lower rate of exacerbations but not directly improve mortality.

93. Shingles (Herpes zoster) is caused by a reactivation of what infection?

Varicella (chicken pox)

94. What agents are the most common cause of food poisoning?

Noroviruses are believed to cause greater than 50% of cases; bacterial causes include *Salmonella* (nontyphoidal), *Campylobacter*, *Clostridium perfringens*, and *Staphylococcus aureus*

95. Sudden death is associated with what cardiac rhythm in patients with prolonged QT syndrome?

Torsades de pointes or ventricular fibrillation

96. For food poisoning, what signs and symptoms should prompt more aggressive care?

In the setting of diarrhea, concerning signs and symptoms include high fever (≥101.3°F), ≥ 6 stools/day, blood in the stools, elevated white blood cell count, signs of dehydration, and diarrheal illness that lasts >2 to 3 days

97. What four muscles make up the rotator cuff?

Supraspinatus
Infraspinatus
Subscapularis
Teres minor (not major)

98. A group of college students develops nausea, vomiting, and diarrhea while traveling to Mexico on spring break. What is the likely diagnosis?

Food poisoning; symptoms can begin within one hour of eating the contaminated food or over 16 hours after exposure.

99. What is the most common genetic disorder in white Americans?

Hereditary hemochromatosis (1 in 250–300 Caucasians are homozygous and 1 in 10 are carriers.)

100. What is the risk of a patient with Barrett esophagitis developing esophageal cancer?

Depending on the degree of dysplasia, somewhere between 0.5 and 6%. Enrollment in a surveillance program dramatically lowers that risk.

101. What is the classic triad of hemochromatosis?

Cutaneous hyperpigmentation
Diabetes mellitus
Cirrhosis (late manifestation)

102. A 19-year-old male presents with diffuse nontender lymphadenopathy in his neck, axilla, and groin and night sweats. His history is significant for mononucleosis at age 14. What condition needs to be ruled out?

Hodgkin lymphoma; having an Epstein-Barr virus infection increases the risk.

103. What are the best initial screening tests for family members of someone with hemochromatosis?

Ferritin and serum transferrin saturation (serum iron concentration divided by TIBC multiplied by 100—normal is 14%–50%)

104. At what ages do patients develop Hodgkin lymphoma?	Hodgkin lymphoma has a bimodal distribution and is most common in early adulthood (15 to 40 years of age) and then again after age 55 years.
105. In patients with cirrhosis, what biochemical marker is used to identify hepatocellular carcinoma?	Alfa fetoprotein
106. Two weeks after returning from a camping trip in rural Maine, a patient develops loose, greasy, foul-smelling stools that tend to float, bloating, and lactose intolerance. What is the likely cause?	Giardia infection can occur following drinking nontreated water. Other risk factors include daycare centers, anal intercourse, wilderness camping, travel to developing countries, children adopted from developing countries, public swimming pools, and pets with Giardia infection/diarrhea.
107. Elevations of B-human chorionic gonadotropin (hCG) is associated with which malignancies?	Liver and germ cell tumors
108. What is the cause of open-angle glaucoma?	Primary open-angle glaucoma (POAG) is an optic neuropathy resulting in visual field loss frequently associated with increased intraocular pressure (IOP) due to impaired aqueous outflow through the trabecular meshwork.
109. What condition is associated with an elevated vanillylmandelic acid (VMA) urine levels?	Pheochromocytoma
110. What is the cause of acute closed-angle glaucoma?	Primary angle-closure suspect (PACS) occurs when the eye has a narrow or occluded anterior chamber angle, but no other abnormalities; it is a medical emergency.

111. At what oxygen level is supplemental oxygen required for flight travel?

Sea-level $PaO_2 < 68$–70 mm Hg

---

112. What are the risk factors for gout?

Age > 40 years, male gender, high-purine diet (meats and seafood), alcohol intake (especially beer), high fructose intake, obesity, hyperuricemia, congestive heart failure, renal disease, organ transplant, metabolic syndrome, diabetes mellitus, and some medications such as thiazide diuretics, loop diuretics, and niacin

---

113. West Nile virus is transmitted by the bite of

Mosquitoes

---

114. How do you discern gout from pseudogout?

Gout has urate crystals that cause negatively birefringent needle-shaped crystals under polarizing microscopy. Pseudogout is due to calcium pyrophosphate dihydrate (CPPD) crystal deposition in the joints that are positively birefringent and are rhomboid shaped.

---

115. Which blood test has the highest specificity for the detection of acute pancreatitis?

Serum lipase
Better than serum amylase, which can be elevated with salivary gland abnormalities

---

116. What are the symptoms of pseudogout?

Acute CPPD disease (pseudogout) presents with pain and swelling of ≥ 1 or more joints; knee involved in 50% of cases; involvement of ankle, wrist, toe, and shoulder is also common. It often involves proximal joints (mimicking polymyalgia rheumatica), and can be accompanied by tibiofemoral and ankle arthritis and tendinous calcifications.

---

117. In polycythemia vera (primary polycythemia), the erythropoietin (EPO) level is

Low
In secondary causes of polycythemia (COPD, renal artery stenosis, renal cell carcinoma, and obstructive sleep apnea), the EPO levels are elevated.

118. What is the most common cause of hyperthyroidism?	Graves disease is an autoimmune disease in which thyroid-stimulating antibodies cause increased thyroid function; classic findings include goiter, ophthalmopathy (orbitopathy), and occasionally dermopathy (pretibial or localized myxedema).
119. According the American Heart Association and the American College of Cardiology, at what level of risk over 10 years should a statin be strongly encouraged?	≥7.5%
120. What are the risk factors for developing Graves disease?	Risk factors for Graves include female gender; childbirth (postpartum period); stressful life events; medications such as iodine, amiodarone, and lithium; highly active antiretroviral treatment (HAART); and smoking.
121. At what low-density lipoprotein (LDL) level, regardless of 10-year risk, should a patient be encouraged to initiate statin therapy?	≥190 mg/dL
122. In patients with known coronary artery disease, current recommendations suggest the LDL goal be less than what level?	70 mg/dL
123. What is Hashimoto thyroiditis?	Hashimoto thyroiditis is an autoimmune destruction of the thyroid gland that can result in progression to overt hypothyroidism and/or goiter formation.
124. What is the most common cause of bacterial diarrhea in the United States?	*Campylobacter*

125. What condition can cause unilateral sensorineural hearing loss with tinnitus and loss of balance?

Acoustic neuroma

126. What tests should be obtained when Hashimoto thyroiditis is suspected?

A TSH should be obtained; if elevated, consider a T4 and a thyroid peroxidase antibody (TPO, an antibody to the thyroid) and a thyroglobulin antibody (TG or TGAb, antibody targets thyroglobulin, the storage form of thyroid hormones).

127. What are the indications for antiviral use in the treatment of influenza?

Antivirals should be started within 48 hours of symptom onset *and* if patient has a condition (i.e., diabetes, coronary heart disease [CHD], COPD, asthma) where risk of complication is great. Antivirals are not indicated in patients at low risk of complication.

128. What are the early symptoms of Huntington disease?

Huntington disease is an autosomal dominant inherited condition that presents in ages 30–50 (after they may have passed it on). Symptoms include:
chorea (nonrepeating, complex, involuntary rhythmic movements);
ballism (sometimes violent, involuntary movements, typically of the upper extremity and unilateral);
tics (repeated spasmodic, typically of the face and upper extremity);
dystonia (movement with persisting spasm);
motor impersistence (inability to sustain a desired movement), myoclonus (sudden, involuntary jerk);
cognitive changes (patients often lack insight into their cognitive deficits);
executive dysfunction; emotional lability; and depression.

129. In a monogamous relationship, what is the lifetime risk of sexual transmission of hepatitis C to an unaffected partner?

<1%
HCV is transmitted through parenteral exposures to contaminated blood, usually through sharing of needles.

130. A 30-year-old female returns with 3 weeks of cough that has been unresponsive to azithromycin and albuterol inhaler; she lets you know that her basement flooded last month and she has been tearing out the carpet. What is her likely diagnosis?

Hypersensitivity pneumonitis; it is a diffuse inflammatory disease of the lung parenchyma caused by an immunologic reaction to aerosolized antigenic particles found in a variety of environments. Initially, it may present with fever, but recurrent exposure can result in prolonged and progressive cough, dyspnea, fatigue, weight loss, could ultimately lead to fibrosis and respiratory failure.

131. How is Hypersensitivity pneumonitis treated?

Decreased exposure to offending agents, oral corticosteroids tapered over 2 weeks, and bronchodilators

132. What category of asthma is classified by daytime symptoms occurring no more than 2 days per week, nighttime symptoms no more than 2 nights per month, and the peak expiratory flow (PEF) or forced expiratory volume in 1 second (FEV_1) is 80% or more of predicted?

Mild intermittent asthma

Internal Medicine

133. An 82-year-old patient presents after passing out; she states she was fine until 3 seconds beforehand she felt "funny." Her husband helped her up quickly, and since she feels fine. What condition is most concerning with a brief prodrome preceding syncope?

A prodrome lasting less than 5 seconds before syncope implies a cardiac arrhythmia and deserves rapid cardiac evaluation. Prodromes lasting more than a few seconds, and associated with nausea or vomiting are likely to have vasovagal syncope.

134. Daytime symptoms occurring more than 2 days per week, but less than once daily, and nighttime symptoms more than two times per month is classified as what category of asthma?

Mild persistent asthma

135. An obese male presents with a persistent numbness over the anterolateral aspect of his thigh with no other associated symptoms. What is the likely diagnosis?

Meralgia paraesthetica is an entrapment of the lateral femoral cutaneous nerve (LFCN). Symptoms include pain, paresthesias, and sensory loss over the anterolateral aspect of the thigh. It is typically caused by a belt or tight-fitting clothes across the lower abdomen. The diagnosis is made clinically by decreased sensation over the anterolateral thigh, and treated by wearing loose clothes, using suspenders, etc.

136. What category of asthma is classified by daytime symptoms occurring daily and nighttime symptoms occurring more than 1 night per week with a PEF or FEV$_1$ 60%–80% of predicted?

Moderate persistent asthma

137. What are the symptoms of narcolepsy?

Narcolepsy is defined as excessive daytime sleepiness often associated with cataplexy (sudden bilateral weakness of skeletal muscles) and other rapid eye movement (REM) sleep phenomena, such as sleep paralysis and hypnagogic hallucinations (e.g., vivid auditory or visual perceptions without an external stimulus that occur as one is falling asleep).

138. Continuous daytime symptoms and frequent nighttime symptoms with a PEF or FEV_1 less than 60% of predicted is classified as what category of asthma?

Severe persistent asthma

139. A 58-year-old male with chronic back pain who uses high doses of NSAIDs presents with peripheral edema; workup finds large proteinuria and new onset hyperlipidemia. What is the likely cause?

Nephrotic syndrome is a clinical syndrome of heavy proteinuria, hypoalbuminemia, hyperlipidemia, and edema.

140. Who should be treated for tuberculosis in recent purified protein derivative converters?

All patients should be treated regardless of age.

141. How is Nephrotic Syndrome treated?

Nephrotic syndrome is treated by salt restriction and salt-wasting diuretics (loop and thiazide diuretics), statins, ACEi or ARBs, and addressing the underlying cause.

142. Why are women usually diagnosed with hemochromatosis at menopause?

Menstrual blood loss (auto-phlebotomy) stops and allows iron overload to occur.

143. An obese patient has an incidentally identified enlarged liver. What condition does obesity induce causing hepatomegaly?

Nonalcoholic fatty liver disease (NAFLD) is due to obesity; the etiology is due to large vacuoles of triglyceride fat accumulate in hepatocytes.

144. For people who received the pneumococcal vaccine (PPSV23) at or after age 65, when should they receive the PCV13 vaccination?

One dose of PCV13 is recommended for all adults 65 years of age or older who have not previously received the vaccine.
For adults 65 years and older who have already received one or more doses of PPSV23, the dose of PCV13 should be given at least 1 year after receiving the most recent dose of PPSV23.

145. How does NAFLD differ from nonalcoholic steatohepatitis (NASH)?

NASH is a progression of NAFLD, but in NASH, liver function tests (LFTs) are elevated and liver biopsy finds fatty deposits in >50% of cells with ballooning, acute/chronic inflammation. In some cases, NASH progresses to cirrhosis and liver failure.

146. Fever and white blood cell (WBC) casts on urinalysis are associated with what condition?

Acute pyelonephritis

147. What causes a painless whitish thickening of the great toe in a 71-year-old man with diabetes?

Onychomycosis, which is a fungal infection of the nails; it predominantly happens on the toes, but can also happen on the hands.

148. Red blood cell casts on urinalysis are associated with what renal abnormality?

Glomerulonephritis

149. What two oral agents increase the risk of avascular necrosis?

Avascular necrosis is associated with chronic corticosteroid use (the dose is cumulative) and alcohol abuse.

150. What is the most common cause of adverse events in hospitalized patients?	Medication-related problems
151. What are the classic findings of cardiac tamponade?	Pericardial effusion/cardiac tamponade presents with Beck triad: hypotension, muffled heart sounds, jugular venous distention.
152. In patients undergoing radiographic procedures that require iodinated contrast, what medication theoretically may increase the risk of lactic acidosis?	Metformin
153. What are the treatment methods for peripheral artery disease (PAD)?	Treating PAD requires an exercise rehabilitation program (walk until symptoms develop, then rest and start again for 30 minutes, then increased by 5 minutes until 50 minutes of intermittent walking is achieved); smoking cessation, weight loss, antiplatelet therapy (aspirin), and statin use.
154. The presence of delta waves with a widened QRS complex and a short PR interval of 0.10 seconds on electrocardiography (ECG) tracings suggest the diagnosis of	Wolff-Parkinson-White (WPW) syndrome
155. What condition would present as a 27-year-old male with weeks of atypical back pain without trauma, burning pain with urination, and conjunctivitis?	Reiter syndrome is a seronegative, multisystem, inflammatory disorder classically involving the joints, the eye, and the lower genitourinary (GU) tract. Axial joints (e.g., spine, sacroiliac joints) are the common presenting complaint. The classic triad includes arthritis, conjunctivitis/iritis, and either urethritis or cervicitis ("can't see; can't pee; can't bend my knee").

156. What is the intravenous (IV) drug of choice for supraventricular tachyarrhythmia (SVT)?

Adenosine

157. A 28-year-old, otherwise healthy male has a persistent nonproductive cough unresponsive to empiric treatment; chest x-ray shows bilateral hilar adenopathy and parenchymal infiltrates. What is the likely cause?

Sarcoidosis; a noninfectious, multisystem granulomatous disease of unknown cause, commonly affecting young and middle-aged adults.
It frequently presents with hilar adenopathy, pulmonary infiltrates, ocular and skin lesions, and in ~50% of cases is diagnosed in asymptomatic patients with abnormal chest x-rays.

158. To screen for peripheral neuropathy, what test is recommended annually to document sensory function in diabetic patients?

Monofilament line test

159. What are the clinical manifestations of Sjogren syndrome?

Sjogren syndrome is a chronic inflammatory disorder resulting in lymphocytic infiltrates in exocrine organs (diminished salivary and lacrimal gland function, resulting in sicca symptoms such as dry eyes (xerophthalmia), dry mouth (xerostomia), and parotid enlargement). Extraglandular manifestations: arthralgia, myalgia, Raynaud phenomenon, pulmonary disease, GI disease, leukopenia, anemia, lymphadenopathy, vasculitis

160. Which class of drugs slows the progression from microalbuminuria to macroalbuminuria (renal protective) in diabetic patients?

ACE inhibitors

161. What are the complications of obstructive sleep apnea?

Obstructive sleep apnea increases the risk of hypertension, stroke, myocardial infarction, diabetes, cardiovascular disease, and work-related and driving accidents.

162. To screen for diabetes-induced nephropathy, what urine test should be checked yearly?

Microalbuminuria

163. What are the symptoms of spinal stenosis?

Spinal stenosis symptoms *worsen with extension* (prolonged standing, walking downhill, or down stairs) and *improve with flexion* (sitting, leaning forward while walking, walking uphill or upstairs, lying in a flexed position).

164. What is the cutoff level of albumin in the urine to be called microalbuminuria?

Urinary albumin of 30–300 mg/day is consistent with microalbuminuria.

If one screening urine is positive, diabetic nephropathy should be confirmed in a total of two out of three samples collected over a 3- to 6-month period because of day-to-day variability.

165. What is SIADH (syndrome of inappropriate antidiuretic hormone secretion)?

A syndrome of abnormal production of antidiuretic hormone (ADH), despite low serum osmolality, leading to hyponatremia and inappropriately elevated urine osmolality. It results in abnormal water retention that leads to dilutional hyponatremia (total body sodium levels may be normal or near normal, but the patient's total body water is increased).

166. In a patient with persistent diarrhea, the presence of a large number of fecal leukocytes is consistent with what?

A bacterial infection

167. What tests should be ordered to rule out von Willebrand disease?

vWF antigen (vWF:Ag), vWF activity/ristocetin cofactor activity (vWF:RCo), and FVIII activity

168. Headaches that are present upon waking but do not interrupt sleep are associated with what condition?

Headaches that are present upon waking may imply increased intracranial pressure. If general, consider tumor; if just occipital and patient has hypertension, consider improving hypertension control.

169. What are the common causes of SIADH?

SIADH can be caused by medications (NSAIDs, others), neurologic disease or trauma, carcinomas, pulmonary conditions, some infections (including HIV), and hypothyroidism.

170. Headaches that appear mid to late afternoon associated with rhinorrhea are commonly caused by what?

Sinus-related inflammation, either from allergic rhinitis or infection

171. What is the treatment of choice for patients diagnosed with *Salmonella enterocolitis*?

Observation
Antibiotics are contraindicated because they tend to prolong the carrier state.

172. What is the pathophysiology of a TIA?

A TIA is a transient episode of neurologic dysfunction due to focal brain, retinal, or spinal cord ischemia without acute infarction.

173. How does having a TIA influence stroke risk?

Having a TIA is the most important predictor of stroke: 7%–40% of patients with stroke report previous TIA.

174. How long does a neurologic deficit have to be present to be considered a TIA?

Any loss of function is considered a TIA; there is no longer a time requirement.

175. What is the treatment of choice for patients with symptomatic iron overload due to hemochromatosis?

Phlebotomy; 500 mL/wk (about 250 mg of iron) until serum iron levels are normal and transferrin saturation is below 50%; 2–6 phlebotomies per year

176. Thiazide diuretics can cause loss of what electrolytes?	Sodium and potassium
177. In patients who are symptomatic from severe hypercalcemia, what is the treatment of choice?	Aggressive fluid administration, followed by loop diuretics, and then calcitonin or bisphosphonates
178. What condition is associated with elevated WBC count and the Philadelphia chromosome?	Chronic myelogenous leukemia is a leukemia with a natural history of three clinical phases: a chronic phase, an accelerated phase, and blast phase or crisis (transformation to acute leukemia).
179. In patients with osteoporosis and hypertension, what class of antihypertensive is beneficial for both conditions?	Thiazide diuretics decrease urine calcium excretion.
180. What are the lifestyle treatments for osteoporosis?	Weightbearing exercise Smoking cessation Physical therapy for muscle strengthening Vitamin D 2,000 IU/day
181. How is osteopenia defined?	The World Health Organization defines osteopenia as a T-score between −1 and −2.5; it should be treated with lifestyle modification (weightbearing exercise, smoking cessation, vitamin D supplementation). Treatments with agents for osteoporosis (bisphosphonates, etc.) are not indicated.
182. How is osteoporosis defined?	On bone mineral density testing, osteoporosis is diagnosed when T-score is ≤2.5.

183. What are the recommended management options for women with atypical squamous cells of undetermined significance (ASC-US)?

Repeat cytology at 12 months (if <25 years) or reflex DNA testing for oncogenic human papillomavirus (HPV) infection types or colposcopy.

184. What is the most commonly involved tendon in shoulder impingement syndrome?

Supraspinatus tendon

185. What is the most common cause of atraumatic shoulder pain in adults?

Impingement syndrome (formerly rotator cuff tendonitis)

186. What is the most common chronic myeloproliferative disorder?

Polycythemia vera

187. What is the international normalized ratio (INR) goal for patients with nonvalvular atrial fibrillation?

2.0–3.0

188. What is the INR goal for patients with artificial cardiac valves?

2.5–3.5

189. What is the INR goal for patients with a deep vein thrombosis (DVT) or pulmonary embolism (PE)?

2.0–3.0

190. What oral dose of vitamin B_{12} is required to effectively treat vitamin B_{12} deficiency?

1–2,000 mg given daily, even with the absence of intrinsic factor (pernicious anemia)

191. What is the most common finding associated with celiac sprue in adults?

Iron deficiency anemia

192. What is the mechanism of action for thiazolidinediones in type 2 diabetes?

Decreasing insulin resistance and decreasing gluconeogenesis
They have no effect on insulin release or production by the pancreas or carbohydrate absorption.
May cause hypoglycemia

193. What is the mechanism of action of polyethylene glycol for constipation?

Osmotic changes in the intestines

194. What is the treatment of choice for cluster headaches?

100% oxygen

195. Noncardiac conditions related to the development of atrial fibrillation include

Hypertension
Diabetes mellitus
COPD
Hyperthyroidism
Primary pulmonary hypertension
Acute PE
Acute ethanol ingestion

196. A headache that consists of at least five severe, recurrent attacks that are unilateral, orbital, supra-orbital, or temporal, causing pain lasting 15–180 minutes if untreated and is associated with conjunctival injection and/or lacrimation, nasal congestion and/or rhinorrhea, eyelid edema, forehead and facial sweating, miosis and/or ptosis, and sense of restlessness or agitation:

Cluster headache

197. Celiac sprue is associated with what food?

Gluten
Found in wheat and rye and cereal protein in barley and oats, but not corn

198. What additional vaccine should those with sickle cell anemia receive?

Pneumococcal vaccine because of decreased ability to fight encapsulated organisms

199. What drug is first-line treatment to prevent a painful sickle cell crisis in those with sickle cell anemia?

Hydroxyurea
Also reduces the incidence of acute chest syndrome and transfusion requirements

200. What is the drug of choice for treating trigeminal neuralgia?

Carbamazepine

201. A headache that is moderate to severe in intensity, located unilaterally, and is associated with an aura, photophobia, nausea, and vomiting is classified as a

Classical migraine headache

202. What is the most serious potential adverse effect of amiodarone therapy?

Pulmonary toxicity

203. Where does the maculopapular erythematous rash associated with Rocky Mountain spotted fever begin?

Petechial rash begins on the extremities (palms and soles) and spreads centrally.

204. In malnourished patients with alcohol abuse, Wernicke encephalopathy is related to a deficiency of

Thiamine coupled with the ingestion of carbohydrates

205. What bone abnormality does celiac sprue predispose patients to?	Osteopenia due to vitamin D deficiency Laboratory values include hypocalcemia and elevated alkaline phosphatase levels.
206. What class of antihypertensive agents is associated with rebound hypertension?	Alpha antagonist (i.e., clonidine)
207. Patients who complain of "clunking" with shoulder range of motion and apprehension when reaching behind their backs are likely to have	Torn labrum of the scapula predisposing patient to dislocation
208. ACE inhibitors are associated with what electrolyte abnormality?	Hyperkalemia—especially in elderly patients with renal disease or those taking β-blockers, nonsteroidal antiinflammatory drugs (NSAIDs), and potassium-sparing diuretics
209. Furosemide use can induce what electrolyte abnormality?	Hypokalemia by enhanced potassium excretion by increasing delivery of sodium to the collecting tubules
210. What condition causes difficulty swallowing associated with chest pain and is due to increased pressure of the lower esophageal sphincter?	Achalasia
211. A patient presents with chest pain with eating and occasionally vomits. You suspect achalasia. What is the most sensitive test for achalasia?	Esophageal manometry

212. A patient presents with an insidious onset of general weakness and fatigue. Examination finds hypotension and hyperpigmentation of the skin and mucous membranes; workup identifies hyponatremia and hyperkalemia. What is the most likely diagnosis?

Primary AI (Addison disease)

213. The cosyntropin stimulation test is used to detect adrenal insufficiency (AI), How is the test conducted?

250 mg of cosyntropin (synthetic analogue of ACTH) is given intravenously or intramuscularly. The serum cortisol is measured 30–60 minutes later. A normal result is a serum cortisol 500 nmol/L. Lower levels suggest the diagnosis of AI.

214. Dexamethasone suppression test is used to diagnose what disease?

Cushing disease (cortisol excess)

215. With iron supplementation, how long does it take for hemoglobin levels to return to a normal level?

Two months
Once ferritin levels have returned to normal, iron replacement can be discontinued.

216. When *Neisseria meningitides* is diagnosed, what antibiotic prophylaxis is necessary for close contacts?

Antibiotic prophylaxis within 24 hours of the diagnosis; treatment options include the following:
Rifampin 600 mg PO BID × 2 days
Ciprofloxacin 500 mg PO × 1 dose
Ceftriaxone 250 mg IM × 1 dose

217. How does the development of congestive heart failure (CHF) in patients with aortic stenosis impact treatment and mortality?

In aortic stenosis and CHF, without valve replacement, 50% will die in 2 years.

218. What is the most common cause of hypercoagulable state?

Factor V Leiden mutation
Other conditions include the following:
Antithrombin III deficiency
Protein C deficiency
Protein S deficiency
Lupus anticoagulant
Antiphospholipid syndrome

219. The presence of spongiform changes (vacuoles in the neurons and glia of the brain) in an individual that develops a rapidly progressive dementia accompanied by myoclonic seizures suggests what diagnosis?

Creutzfeldt-Jakob disease

220. What tests should be followed for patients taking amiodarone?

Liver and thyroid function tests should be monitored at least every 6 months.

221. An S4 gallop is heard just before normal heart sounds and is associated with what conditions?

S4 gallop is associated with poor ventricular compliance (increased stiffness of the ventricle) due to left ventricular hypertrophy (hypertensive heart disease), aortic stenosis, heart failure, or acute myocardial infarction (MI)

222. What is the infectious cause of posttransfusion hepatitis infections?

Hepatitis C

223. What medication is indicated for the treatment of acute pericarditis?

NSAIDs

224. What diagnostic test can be used to detect hepatitis B in the "window period" (the period between the presence of hepatitis B surface antigen and the development of hepatitis B surface antibody)?

IgM hepatitis B core antibody (IgM anti-HBc)

225. According to the USPSTF, who should be screened for hepatitis C?

Offer one-time screening for hepatitis C virus (HCV) infection to adults born between 1945 and 1965 and those at high risk for infection (hemodialysis, tattoo in unregulated setting, blood/blood product transfusion or organ transplantation before 1992, hemophilia treatment before 1987, exposure to infected body fluids, history of incarceration, children born to HCV-positive mothers, current sexual partners of HCV-positive persons, any history of injection drug use, intranasal illicit drug use, and HIV or hepatitis B infection).

226. What is Hepatitis D?

Hepatitis D virus or delta agent
It is a serologic marker associated with an unusually severe acute infection with hepatitis B. It is a defective RNA virus that replicates only in the presence of hepatitis B virus and represents a coinfection and is especially seen in illicit drug users.

227. What infection is associated with ingesting contaminated raw milk products?

Brucellosis is transmitted via contact with secretions or excretions of infected animals or ingesting raw milk or products of raw milk.

228. Clear, watery stools with a fishy odor and flecks of mucus (rice water diarrhea) are in what conditions?

Cholera and shigella

229. What infectious disease affects hunters, butchers, fur handlers, and farmers who harvest wild rabbit fur?

Tularemia
The organism may be found in skin lesions.

230. What conditions can induce erectile dysfunction?

Diabetes, vascular problems, prolactinoma, hypothyroidism, testosterone deficiency
The most common cause is psychological, which is likely if the patient has morning erections.

231. Visual flashes of light (photopsia), associated with the sudden appearance of floaters, and/or peripheral visual field loss suggest what diagnosis?	Retinal detachment
232. Vitreous detachment (separation of the vitreous from the retina) may lead to what dangerous eye condition?	Retinal detachment
233. What vitamin is used to correct elevations in INR values secondary to warfarin use?	Parenteral vitamin K
234. What classes of medications should all CHF patients be on, if not contraindicated?	Aspirin ACE inhibitor β-Blocker For those with Class II–IV, loop diuretics and potassium-sparing diuretics
235. What potentially life-threatening condition affecting the mucous membranes and airways is associated with the use of ACE inhibitors?	Angioneurotic edema
236. Bulimia induces what electrolyte abnormalities?	Hypokalemia and metabolic alkalosis
237. What are common secondary causes of resistant hypertension?	Most common secondary causes of resistant hypertension are obstructive sleep apnea, renal artery stenosis, renal parenchymal disease, and primary aldosteronism.

238. What is the most common type of lung cancer?

Non–small cell lung cancer is the most common, making up 85% of primary lung malignancies. These lesions typically begin at the periphery. Subtypes include adenocarcinoma, squamous cell lung cancer, and large cell carcinoma.

239. What are the clinical symptoms of periodic limb movement disorder?

Periodic limb movement disorders is characterized by periodic repetitive limb movements during sleep, typically of the lower extremities, and associated with sleep disturbance and arousal, which can lead to sleep disruption and ultimately daytime sleepiness.

240. What are the four cardinal features of restless legs syndrome (RLS)?

The four cardinal features of RLS are
1. an urge to move the limbs often associated with paresthesias or dysesthesias
2. symptom onset or becoming worse with inactivity
3. some relief of symptoms with movement
4. worsening of symptoms in the evening or at night

241. What is a normal postvoid residual of the bladder?

A normal postvoid residual volume is less than 50 mL.

242. What oral and dental clues are consistent with bulimia?

Eroded dental enamel, dental caries, angular cheilitis, gingivitis, and swollen salivary glands

243. What electrolyte abnormality can be caused by both selective serotonin reuptake inhibitors (SSRIs) and serotonin–norepinephrine reuptake inhibitors (SNRIs)?

Hyponatremia

244. What condition occurs when patients on chronic opioid treatment develop painful sensitivity to skin pressure?

Opioid-induced hyperalgesia
It is treated by lowering the opioid dose.

245. When treating stroke, thrombolytics must be administered within what time frame from the onset of stroke-related symptoms?

180 minutes (3 hours)

246. A patient without a spleen should have what intervention whenever he or she develops a fever?

All patients who are asplenic should have antibiotics prescribed whenever they have a fever.

247. What immunizations should patients receive if they are asplenic?

Both pneumococcal conjugate vaccine (PCV13) and pneumococcal polysaccharide vaccine (PPSV23) should be given at least 8 weeks apart as well as the influenza vaccine each year.

248. Define chronic bronchitis.

Chronic bronchitis is associated with excessive cough and sputum production on most days for at least 3 months during 2 consecutive years.

249. Based on 2014 JNC VIII guidelines, what drugs should be used first line in the general nonblack population for essential hypertension?

For nonblack adults, including those with diabetes, initial treatment should include a thiazide-type diuretic, calcium-channel blocker (CCB), ACE inhibitor, or angiotensin receptor blocker (ARB).

250. What are contraindications to the use of ACE inhibitors?

History of angioneurotic edema, pregnancy, and renal artery stenosis

251. According to the 2014 JNC VIII guidelines, what drugs are first choice for the black population?

In the general black population, including those with diabetes, initial treatment should include a thiazide-type diuretic or a CCB.

252. What type of ultraviolet exposure is associated with skin cancer?

Ultraviolet B (UVB)

253. What BMI is consistent with obesity?

$\geq 30 \text{ kg/m}^2$

Internal Medicine

254. What weight loss medication is associated with flatus, oily stools, and diarrhea?

Orlistat (Xenical)

255. What is the cause of a tremor that affects the hands and forearms when the limb is voluntarily moved and/or when held against gravity?

Essential tremor is a postural (occurring with voluntary maintenance of a position against gravity) or kinetic (occurring during voluntary movement) flexion–extension tremor that is slow and rhythmic and primarily affects the hands and forearms, head, and voice.

256. What medications are used for control of essential tremors?

Propranolol or primidone

257. What percentage of diarrheal cases in the United States are not associated with an identifiable pathogen?

More than 50%

258. What condition is associated with lytic lesions of the bone, hypercalcemia, and increased infection risk?

Multiple myeloma. It is a clonal proliferation of malignant plasma cells in the bone marrow that can cause osteolytic lesions and pathologic fractures. The malignant plasma cells produce monoclonal Bence Jones protein in the blood and urine.

259. What condition can cause a lytic lesion on a plain x-ray but have a normal bone scan?

Multiple myeloma will not be seen on a conventional bone scan.

260. The presence of proteinuria and lytic bone lesions should suggest what diagnosis?

Multiple myeloma

261. A progressive destructive arthritis secondary to peripheral neuropathy and the associated loss of pain in a diabetic is called

Charcot foot

262. A rapidly growing dome-shaped lesion with a central umbilication is likely a

Keratoacanthoma

263. What selective estrogen receptor modulator (SERM) is used to treat osteoporosis and can lower the risk of breast cancer?

Raloxifene (Evista)
Its common side effects include hot flushes and leg cramps.

264. How does a vegan diet differ from a vegetarian diet?

Vegans will not use any animal products (eggs, milk, and milk products). Some vegans also will not use leather and wool.

265. Herpes simplex virus type 1 (HSV-1) traditionally affects what region of the body?

HSV-1 traditionally presents with blisters on lips and in mouth, face, and eyes.

266. A patient who develops a low-grade fever, myalgias, headache, tachycardia, and rash shortly after the first dose of doxycycline for Lyme disease has what condition?

Jarisch-Herxheimer reaction

267. Digoxin needs to be dosed carefully in patients with what organ deficiency?

Kidney disease
Digoxin is primarily excreted through the kidneys; only about 10% is metabolized by the liver.

268. What drug is used for digoxin toxicity?

Digoxin-specific antibody fragments (Digibind)

269. Runners who develop lateral knee pain related to running on uneven surfaces are likely to have

Iliotibial band (ITB) syndrome

270. What condition is associated with tinnitus, hearing loss, and vertigo?

Meniere disease

271. What medications are used for the treatment of Meniere disease?

Thiazide diuretics such as hydrochlorothiazide, and antiemetics

272. Which test is commonly used to confirm systemic lupus erythematosus (SLE)?

Anti–double-stranded DNA test

273. What condition is associated with idiopathic intermittent episodes of vasoconstriction of digital arteries, in response to cold, emotional stress, or blunt trauma?

Raynaud phenomenon

274. What class of medication is used to control the symptoms of Raynaud phenomenon?

Calcium-channel blockers (nifedipine and diltiazem)

275. What condition is the most common risk factor for the development of acute respiratory distress syndrome (ARDS)?

Sepsis (especially from an abdominal source)

276. Polydipsia, polyphagia, polyuria, weight loss, and fatigue are among the presenting symptoms of what diagnosis?

Type 1 diabetes mellitus

277. Chronic acid exposure to the lower esophagus that causes a transformation of squamous to columnar epithelium is called	Barrett's esophagus
278. Presence of elevated serum carboxyhemoglobin levels is associated with what condition?	Carbon monoxide poisoning
279. What is the treatment for acute carbon monoxide poisoning?	100% oxygen administration
280. What functional intestinal disorder is associated with abdominal pain, a change in bowel habits, and no organic process?	Irritable bowel syndrome It can present as diarrhea predominant or constipation predominant; initial treatments include fiber supplements and antispasmodics.
281. What area of induration is considered positive on a Mantoux tuberculin skin test?	An area of induration of >15 mm (without risk factors) An area of induration of >10 mm (with risk factors) An area of induration of > 5 mm (in HIV patients)
282. What activity results in the single largest health risk in the United States?	Smoking
283. What class of antihypertensive medications slows progression of renal disease in diabetes mellitus?	ACE inhibitors If patient cannot tolerate an ACE inihibitor, an ARB may be used.
284. A painless ulcer that develops on the genitals is consistent with what sexually transmitted infection (STI)?	Syphilis A skin lesion that begins as a papule that ruptures and develops into a painless ulcer is called a chancre.

285. What tests are used to screen for syphilis?

Venereal Disease Research Laboratory (VDRL) and rapid plasma reagin (RPR) tests

286. When a patient has a positive VDRL or RPR test, what test should be ordered to confirm the diagnosis of syphilis?

Fluorescent treponemal antibody absorption test

287. What is the most common etiology of adults with chronic cough?

Postnasal drip

288. Which class of antihypertensives is associated with cough?

ACE inhibitors

289. What is the most common cell type of testicular tumor?

Seminoma

290. Cryptorchidism is associated with what condition?

Testicular tumors

291. Carpal-pedal spasms, anxiety, and circumoral paresthesias are associated with what condition?

Hyperventilation

292. How is orthostatic hypotension diagnosed?

Blood pressure determination when supine and standing, with a decrease in systolic blood pressure of at least 20 mm Hg and in diastolic blood pressure of at least 10 mm Hg

293. What is the condition that occurs within days to weeks following an MI that causes chest pain, fever, pleurisy, pleural effusions, and joint pain called?

Postmyocardial infarction syndrome (or Dressler syndrome)

Internal Medicine

294. A chronic inflammatory syndrome associated with dry mouth, dry eyes (keratoconjunctivitis sicca), dryness of other mucous membranes, and arthritis is	Sjogren syndrome
295. What are the clinical states requiring placement of a permanent pacemaker?	Symptomatic bradycardia, asymptomatic Mobitz II atrioventricular (AV) block, and complete heart block
296. What clinical syndrome characterized by pain and morning stiffness of the shoulder, hip girdles, and neck in patients over age 50 is associated with a vasculitis?	Polymyalgia rheumatica. It is associated with giant cell (temporal) arteritis.
297. What is the treatment of choice for polymyalgia rheumatica?	Corticosteroids (high dose)
298. Aspirin is used for primary prevention of what two conditions?	Colon cancer and atherosclerotic cardiovascular disease
299. A herpes zoster infection that affects the facial nerve is called	Ramsay Hunt syndrome It is a herpes zoster infection of the facial nerve's geniculate ganglion.
300. What is the first-line therapy for the treatment of mild *Clostridium difficile*?	Metronidazole For infections unresponsive to metronidazole or severe infections, oral vancomycin is used.
301. What test should be performed after finding a positive Mantoux test?	Chest x-ray should be done before initiating treatment to exclude active tuberculosis.

302. What intervention is as effective as medication for mild to moderate depression?

Cognitive behavioral therapy

303. To prevent decompression illness, how long should a diver wait to fly after scuba diving?

12 hours

304. What is erysipelas?

Erysipelas is a cellulitis notable for acute, well-demarcated, superficial bacterial skin infection with lymphatic involvement almost always caused by *Streptococcus pyogenes* in infants, children, and adults >40 years; the incidence is greatest in the elderly (>75 years).

305. In patients with chronic abdominal pain and a negative laboratory and clinical exam, what condition should be screened for?

Domestic violence, past or present; history of sexual abuse

306. With right upper quadrant abdominal pain that worsens after meals and normal liver function tests (LFTs) and ultrasound, what test should be considered to rule out biliary dysfunction?

HIDA Scan (hepatobiliary scintigraphy or hepatobiliary iminodiacetic acid scan)

307. What is the drug of choice to treat acetaminophen overdose?

N-acetylcysteine (NAC)

308. What conditions are commonly associated with a low-MCV anemia?

Iron-deficiency anemia, thalassemia, lead poisoning, hemoglobinopathies, sideroblastic anemia

309. What conditions are included in a Wells Score to determine risk of DVT?

One point each for cancer, calf swelling >3 cm, collateral vein engorgement, pitting edema, previous DVT, venous pain, recent immobilization (cast, paralysis), recent bedriddenness
Subtract 2 points if any other diagnosis is likely.

310. What is vertigo that comes on with head movement, lasting just seconds to minutes, associated with rotary nystagmus during Dix-Hallpike maneuver?

Benign paroxysmal positional vertigo (BPPV)

311. How is BPPV treated?

Epley's maneuver

312. What is the first step in evaluating hyponatremia?

Obtain serum osmolality: if >280 mEq/L, it is likely pseudohyponatremia due to hyperlipidemia, hyperglycemia, or hyperproteinemia. If <280 mEq/L, obtain a urinary sodium test.

313. What are the likely causes of hyponatremia with serum osmolality <280 mEq/L and an elevated urine sodium?

Hypothyroidism, syndrome of inappropriate antidiuretic hormone secretion, thiazide diuretics, central nervous system disease, Addison disease

314. Knee pain and swelling that begin without trauma and within a few days of new activity, and pain with going down stairs is likely

Meniscus injury

315. Preoperative evaluation for noncardiac surgery in an adult without cardiovascular disease and ability to walk up a flight of stairs without symptoms (equivalent to 4 METS) include which tests?

None
Labs and ECGs are no longer indicated.

316. Impingement syndrome of the shoulder affects which tendon most frequently?

Supraspinatus tendon
The other tendons of the rotator cuff are infra-spinatus, teres minor, and subscapularis.

317. According to the USPSTF, who should be screened for abdominal aortic aneurysm?

Men aged 65–75 who have ever smoked should receive a one-time abdominal ultrasound.

318. What is a idiopathic inflammatory condition affecting *just* the colonic mucosa, associated with large joint arthritic conditions, sacroiliitis, and ankylosing spondylitis?

Ulcerative colitis

319. What is a chronic relapsing inflammatory disorder that can affect the entire GI tract, causes transmural lesions that skip areas, and can increase the risk of GI cancer?

Crohn disease

320. What can cause shoulder pain that has an insidious onset, has been present for months, and initially had pain only with active range of motion (ROM) but now has pain with both active and passive ROM?

Adhesive capsulitis ("frozen shoulder")

Internal Medicine

321. A patient's bilirubin is mildly elevated; on repeat, it remains so and is unconjugated. The hemoglobin and hematocrit (H&H) is normal, as are the rest of the LFTs. What is the likely diagnosis?	Gilbert syndrome is mild, chronic, or intermittent unconjugated hyperbilirubinemia (not due to hemolysis) with otherwise normal liver function.
322. What is the likely cause of jaundice in a patient with a direct bilirubin <0.3 mg/dL and whose alkaline phosphatase is normal?	Prehepatic jaundice from hemolytic anemia or resorption of a large hematoma
323. An obese patient presents with rash about the neck that is composed of symmetric, hyperpigmented, hyperkeratotic, velvety to verrucous brown plaques. What is the diagnosis?	Acanthosis nigricans due to hyperinsulinemia, often due to uncontrolled diabetes Rash can also occur at flexural and intertriginous surfaces (axilla, elbow, inframammary areas, groin, and anogenital regions).
324. What is the likely diagnosis of a sudden, diffuse hair loss that occurs 2–6 months after a major stressor?	Telogen effluvium
325. Treatment of telogen effluvium includes what patient education?	Reassurance that the hair will regrow within a few months. No other intervention is recommended.
326. What treatments are available for male-pattern hair loss (androgenic alopecia)?	Minoxidil (Rogaine), finasteride (Propecia), and spironolactone

327. What tests should be obtained if anabolic steroid use is suspected?

Urine testosterone: epitestosterone (T:E) ratio (T:E ratio >3:1 suggests anabolic-androgenic steroid abuse)

Serum: Lipids (LDL increase, high-density lipoprotein [HDL] decrease) and LFT elevations (AST, ALT, and GGTP)

---

328. What visual fields are affected by glaucoma?

Glaucoma affects *peripheral* vision, causing tunnel vision.

---

329. A 25-year-old male has 5 months of back pain that gets worse when supine and has morning back stiffness that takes an hour to improve. What is the likely diagnosis?

Ankylosing spondylitis

---

330. A patient who has recently returned from the topics has a high fever (104°F), anemia, diffuse myalgias and is anemic. What is the likely diagnosis?

Dengue hemorrhagic fever presents as a flulike illness, with high fever (104°F) and at least two additional symptoms: severe anemia or hemorrhage, retroorbital pain, myalgias/arthralgias, nausea/vomiting, adenopathy, and rash. It is thought to be an antibody reaction to a different serotype of dengue than prior exposure.

---

331. Painful ovoid or round ulcerations on the mucous membranes of the mouth and tongue are called

Aphthous ulcers or canker sores
Treatment is symptomatic.

---

332. What clinical finding differentiates Zika virus from Dengue fever?

Conjunctivitis; Zika and dengue share the other common symptoms of fever, myalgia, joint pain, retroocular pain, and maculopapular rash.

---

333. What is the difference between Cushing syndrome and Cushing disease?

Cushing syndrome is the result of excess glucocorticoids; Cushing disease is due to excess ACTH production, most commonly from a pituitary adenoma.

---

334. What are the universal findings in a patient with fibromyalgia?

Chronic bilateral, widespread pain $\geq$ 3 months involving limbs and axial skeleton, and fatigue with sleep disturbance

335. What tests should be performed on a patient with alarm symptoms for peptic ulcer disease (episodic gnawing or burning epigastric pain, pain occurring after meals or on empty stomach, and nocturnal pain)?

If peptic ulcer is suspected by history, rectal exam for heme testing should be done, followed by *H. pylori* testing (breath urea or stool antigen; serum antibody testing is inconsistent), and esophagogastroduodenoscopy (EGD) if risk factors exist.

336. What are the laboratory findings of acute Graves disease?

Suppressed (low) TSH with an elevated T4; the next step in the evaluation is to obtain a radioactive iodine uptake (RAIU) scan. Patients with Graves disease will have diffuse, elevated RAIU (vs. localized/nodular elevated uptake in adenoma and multinodular goiter and a decreased uptake in thyroiditis or exogenous thyroid hormone)

337. What are the symptoms of Hashimoto thyroiditis?

Early in the disease, patients may present with symptoms of hyperthyroidism including palpitation, weight loss, and tremors. However, most patients present with symptoms of hypothyroidism including fatigue, cold intolerance, mild weight gain, hoarse voice, dry skin, hair loss, brittle nails, constipation, menstrual irregularity, galactorrhea, and decreased libido.

338. A headache that consists of at least five severe, recurrent attacks that are unilateral, orbital, supraorbital, or temporal, causing pain lasting 15–180 minutes if untreated and is associated with conjunctival injection and/or lacrimation, nasal congestion and/or rhinorrhea, eyelid edema, forehead and facial sweating, miosis and/or ptosis, and sense of restlessness or agitation:

Cluster headache

339. What hepatitis vaccine is recommended for travelers to endemic areas where the infectious agent is associated with fecal to oral transmission?

Hepatitis A

340. What cardiac conditions are indications for ACE inhibitors?

MI and CHF

341. What type of lung cancer begins centrally and is very aggressive?

Small cell carcinoma (previously called oat cell carcinoma)

342. Use of anorectic medication for obesity is acceptable when the BMI is

Greater than 30 kg/m^2 or 27 kg/m^2 with co-morbidities such as hypertension or diabetes mellitus

343. What conditions are commonly associated with an elevated-MCV anemia?

B_{12} deficiency, folate deficiency, alcohol abuse, liver disease, chronic blood loss (menorrhagia, etc.).

344. What test should be ordered with a low-probability Wells Score (–2 to 0) to rule out DVT?

When risk is low, order a d-dimer test. When risk is intermediate (Wells score 1–2), order a high-sensitivity d-dimer; when high (Wells score >2), obtain d-dimer and venous duplex ultrasound.

345. According to the USPSTF, at what ages should women be screened for cervical cancer?

Women age 21–65 years with cytology (Pap smear) every 3 years or, for women age 30–65 years who want to lengthen the screening interval, screening with a combination of cytology and HPV testing every 5 years

3 Obstetrics and Gynecology

1. What anticoagulant medication is generally avoided during pregnancy?

Warfarin (Coumadin)—warfarin is a teratogen and can cross the placenta to cause fetal bleeding and hemorrhagic death of fetus.

2. A healthy 32-year-old female is found to have secondary infertility. She has developed worsened premenstrual symptoms (PMS) since her pregnancy and now has dyspareunia. Laparoscopy finds growths on the ovaries and peritoneal surfaces. What is the likely cause?

Endometriosis: estrogen-dependent implants of endometrial tissue found outside the uterus. Endometriomas are most commonly seen in the peritoneum (bladder, cul-de-sac, pelvic wall, ligaments, ovaries, fallopian tubes, and rectovaginal septum) as well as liver, bowel, umbilicus, and lung.

3. What is used for pregnant women with antiphospholipid syndrome but have never had an adverse outcome related to the condition?

Low-dose aspirin

4. What is the differential diagnosis for galactorrhea?

Pituitary adenoma, pregnancy-induced lactation or recent weaning, nonmilky nipple discharge, intraductal papilloma, fibrocystic disease; if purulent breast discharge, consider mastitis, breast abscess, impetigo, eczema. If bloody breast discharge, consider malignancy.

5. How should women with antiphospholipid antibody syndrome and history of early miscarriages be treated to prevent miscarriage?

Either 81 mg ASA alone or in combination with low molecular weight heparin (LMWH)

6. A young woman is obese and has hirsutism. What laboratory outcomes are associated with polycystic ovary syndrome (PCOS)?

LH: FSH ratio > 2.5:1
Hyperglycemia/insulin resistance
Elevated testosterone levels
Normal prolactin levels (elevated prolactin may imply a pituitary tumor causing PCOS-like syndrome)

---

7. A 19-year-old female has lower abdominal pain for the last 8 days without fever; urine hCG is negative. On exam, she has pain with cervical range of motion and white discharge from the os. What is the likely cause?

Pelvic inflammatory disease (PID); Centers for Disease Control and Prevention (CDC) recommend empiric treatment for PID if one or more of the following minimum criteria are present on pelvic exam in an at-risk patient: cervical motion tenderness, uterine tenderness, and adnexal tenderness in the presence of lower abdominal or pelvic pain.

---

8. What condition is associated with a decreased alfa fetoprotein level?

Down syndrome

---

9. Emergency contraception is most efficacious when it is given within what time frame?

As early as possible, and best within 72 hours

---

10. How does emergency contraception influence an existing pregnancy?

Emergency contraception does not interfere with an existing pregnancy (i.e., patient was raped and presents for emergency contraception but was unknowingly pregnant weeks before the rape). Emergency contraception also does not cause fetal malformations.

---

11. What is the most accurate measure of gestational age in the second or third trimester?

Biparietal diameter, the transverse diameter of fetal head on ultrasound

---

12. What is the leading cause of congenital hearing loss?

Cytomegalovirus (CMV)

13. What are the long-term sequelae of having contracted PID?

A history of PID infection increases the risk of infertility, ectopic pregnancy, and recurrence of infection.

14. What is the most common cause of urinary tract infections in pregnant females?

Escherichia coli

15. What risk is increased in a pregnant woman with asymptomatic bacteriuria?

Increased risk of preterm delivery

16. Preterm labor is defined as

Regular contractions with cervical change before 37 weeks of gestation

17. In women with recurrent pregnancy loss, what coagulation disorder should be tested for?

Antiphospholipid antibody syndrome

18. PCOS is associated with what clinical manifestations?

Menstrual irregularities: oligomenorrhea or amenorrhea
Hyperandrogenism: hirsutism, acne
Insulin resistance: obesity, diabetes mellitus type 2

19. What drug can be used safely in the treatment of Graves disease during first trimester of pregnancy?

Propylthiouracil (PTU)
However, recent guidelines recommend transitioning PTU to methimazole in the second trimester, as the risk of hepatotoxicity in PTU outweighs the teratogenic effect on organogenesis in the first trimester by methimazole.

20. A woman develops painless vaginal bleeding at 36 weeks of pregnancy; what is the greatest worry?

Placenta previa presents with painless bleeding during the second and third trimesters. Placenta previa is when placental tissue extends over or lies proximate to the internal os. Complete/total previa: Placenta covers the entire os. Partial previa: Placenta covers part of internal cervical os.

21. Why is methimazole generally NOT used in the first trimester for the treatment of Graves disease during pregnancy?

Methimazole is associated with congenital abnormalities, and can cross the placenta to induce hypothyroidism in the fetus if not dosed correctly.

22. What are the clinical benefits of raloxifene?

Raloxifene is a selective estrogen receptor modulator (SERM) that acts as an estrogen antagonist in the breast and uterus, but has agonist activity on bone.

As a result, it is used in breast cancer treatment and prevention as well as postmenopausal osteoporosis.

No increased risk in endometrial cancer (as opposed to tamoxifen) but it does increase risk of deep vein thrombosis (DVT).

23. Tamoxifen can increase the risk of what malignancy?

Endometrial carcinoma; tamoxifen is an estrogen antagonist in the breast but has agonist activity in the uterus.

24. When should cervical cancer screening be started, and repeated?

At age 21 years
Repeat:
- If 21–24 years and human papillomavirus (HPV) negative, repeat in 3 years
- If 25–30 years and HPV negative, repeat every 3 years
- If ≥30 years and HPV negative, repeat every 5 years

25. What is the danger of using trimethoprim/sulfamethoxazole (Bactrim/Septra) in the third trimester of pregnancy?

Kernicterus. Sulfonamides can displace bilirubin from albumin and lead to elevated unconjugated bilirubin levels.

26. Recommended management options for women 21–24 years with atypical squamous cells of undetermined significance (ASC-US) include

Reflex DNA testing for oncogenic HPV types
Or
Repeat cytology in 12 months

27. Define metrorrhagia.

Bleeding occurring at irregular intervals, typically *between* normal menstrual cycles

28. Define menometrorrhagia.

Heavy or prolonged bleeding occurring at irregular, noncyclic intervals

29. What position should pregnant women be advised to sleep in?

Pregnant women should be advised to lie in the left lateral decubitus position because the uterus can compress the great vessels, resulting in decreased uterine blood flow.

30. Name the clinical benefits to using oral contraceptives.

Decreased risk of endometrial and ovarian carcinoma (benefit occurs with 1 year of use)
Reduction in dysfunctional uterine bleeding (DUB), menorrhagia, and dysmenorrhea
Improvement in acne, hirsutism
Improved pelvic pain secondary to endometriosis

31. What are the 2015 FDA classifications on medications used during pregnancy?

FDA issued new drug labeling guidelines that remove the product letter categories A, B, D, X. The new system has three categories: pregnancy, lactation, and females and males of reproductive potential. Risk summary, clinical considerations, and data are described for each category.

32. How frequently should women with a hysterectomy for noncancerous reasons receive a pap smear?

Further pap smears are *not* necessary.

33. A patient with symptoms of galactorrhea and has an elevated prolactin level. The next appropriate test is

MRI of the pituitary with gadolinium enhancement

34. What are the clinical findings consistent with congenital rubella syndrome?	Cardiac: patent ductus arteriosus, pulmonary artery stenosis Ophthalmologic: cataracts, retinopathy, glaucoma Neurologic: behavioral disorders, meningoencephalitis, mental retardation Auditory: sensorineural hearing loss Hematologic: thrombocytopenia (petechiae and purpura), hyperbilirubinemia
35. For patients to be diagnosed with bacterial vaginosis, what are the Amsel criteria?	1. pH > 4.5 (most sensitive) 2. Clue cells > 20% (most specific) 3. Homogenous, thin, grayish white discharge 4. Positive whiff test (amine odor with KOH application) Patients should test positive for three out of four to make the diagnosis.
36. Epidurals in delivery are associated with what adverse effects?	Increased duration of second stage of labor and increased risk of maternal fever
37. PCOS is associated with which conditions?	Endometrial carcinoma Infertility Chronic oligomenorrhea/amenorrhea in PCOS leads to decreased progesterone and unopposed increase in estrogen.
38. What are the risk factors for endometrial cancer?	Excessive and unopposed estrogen exposure Tamoxifen therapy Obesity Late menopause Diabetes mellitus Nulliparity Hypertension (HTN)
39. Contraindications to combination oral contraceptives include	A history of venous thromboembolism, stroke, cardiovascular disease, or peripheral vascular disease Smoking if age 35 or over and ≥ 15 cigarettes/day is a relative contraindication. Active liver disease Estrogen-dependent cancers Untreated HTN (controlled HTN is not)

40. Define fetal macrosomia.

Macrosomia is when a fetus weighs more than 4,000 g. Fetal macrosomia is no longer an indication for induction or cesarean section.

41. What biochemical marker is most clinically useful at identifying impending preterm delivery?

Fetal fibronectin in cervical or vaginal secretions helps identify impending preterm delivery.

42. What is the risk of leaving a diaphragm in place for more than 24 hours?

Toxic shock syndrome

43. Painful lesions or nodules found on the shins of women taking birth control pills or newly pregnant:

These nodules are consistent with erythema nodosum. This condition can also occur in inflammatory bowel disease, sarcoidosis, Behcet syndrome, multiple other conditions (strep infections, mononucleosis, hepatitis C), and with the use of multiple medications (sulfonamides, omeprazole, bromides).

44. What biochemical marker is useful in detecting ectopic pregnancy at 5 weeks' gestation?

Serum hCG level
Serum hCG should double every 72 hours in a viable pregnancy; in ectopic pregnancies and nonviable intrauterine pregnancies, hCG levels will plateau or rise but at a slower rate.

45. What embryonic or fetal finding is detectable when the hCG level is 17,000 mIU/mL?

Cardiac activity can be detected.
> 1,000 mIU/mL: a gestational sac can be visualized in the uterus (usually 5 weeks' gestation).
> 2,500 mIU/mL; yolk sac is visible.
> 5,000 mIU/mL: usually the fetal pole can be detected.

46. Vaccines that are safe to provide during pregnancy include

Tdap
Hepatitis B vaccine
Influenza vaccine
Meningococcal vaccine
Rabies vaccine

Obstetrics and Gynecology

47. What clinical signs and symptoms imply an inevitable pregnancy loss?	Inevitable abortion: bleeding, open os, impending passage of product of conception
48. What signs and symptoms imply an incomplete abortion?	Incomplete abortion: bleeding, open os, some passage of products of conception in os or vagina
49. What signs and symptoms imply a threatened abortion?	Threatened abortion: bleeding, closed os, no products of conception in os or vagina; fetus still in utero and viable
50. What signs and symptoms imply a completed abortion?	A completed abortion: bleeding, closed os, complete passage of products of conception on ultrasound. A missed abortion: mild bleeding or cramping, closed os. Loss of early pregnancy symptoms like nausea or breast tenderness, but can also be asymptomatic. Embryo or fetus still present on ultrasound, but no longer viable.
51. What are the main signs and symptoms of septic abortion?	Fever, signs of sepsis, foul smelling vaginal discharge, bleeding, and abdominal pain
52. What increases the risk of a septic abortion?	Induced abortions are more likely to lead to septic abortion than spontaneous abortions.
53. A pregnant patient in the first trimester presents with vaginal bleeding. What are your next management steps?	Pelvic exam should be done to assess cervical os opening and signs of spontaneous abortion, ultrasound, and hCG levels. Spotting can be normal in early pregnancy but vaginal bleeding in the first trimester is ectopic pregnancy until proven otherwise.
54. What are the major complications associated with retained products of conception?	Coagulopathy and infection Patient should get repeat ultrasound after initial management to confirm products of conception are all gone.

55. Besides early sexual activity and multiple partners, what behavior increases the risk of cervical cancer?

Smoking

56. What are the clinical findings associated with HELLP syndrome?

HELLP syndrome is a potentially life threatening complication of late pregnancy that may be a variant of pre-eclampsia. It is associated with Right Upper Quadrant pain and the following:
Hemolysis
Elevated liver enzymes
Low platelets
Right upper quadrant (RUQ) pain

57. A 38-year-old female presents with acute left lower quadrant (LLQ) abdominal pain and you are concerned about an ovarian torsion. What test will help make the diagnosis?

Ultrasound with color Doppler

58. What antibiotics are contraindicated during pregnancy?

Trimethoprim/sulfamethoxazole can cause kernicterus.
Fluoroquinolones can affect cartilage development.
Tetracyclines can affect growth and staining of teeth.

59. Define the first stage of labor.

Time from the start of regular contractions to complete dilation of the cervix

60. What marks the beginning and the end of the second stage of labor?

Time between complete dilation of the cervix to delivery of the baby

61. What class of antihypertensive medications is contraindicated in all stages of pregnancy?

Angiotensin converting enzyme (ACE) inhibitors

62. What antihypertensive medications are considered safe during pregnancy?

Long-acting nifedipine
Labetolol
Thiazide diuretics
Methyldopa

63. When treating eclampsia with magnesium sulfate, what physical exam finding is lost?

Deep tendon reflexes

64. When should screening for *Chlamydia* be instituted?

Screen all sexually active women age 24 years and younger and in older women who are at increased risk.

65. A pregnant woman at 38 weeks has vaginal bleeding. What test should be ordered on vaginal secretions to discern maternal vs fetal blood?

The Apt test is used to discern if the source of late pregnancy bleeding is the infant's or the mother's blood.

66. What are the risk factors for pre-eclampsia?

Nulliparity; age >40 years; family history of preeclampsia; high body mass index; diabetes; chronic HTN, chronic renal disease, or both; multifetal pregnancy; previous preeclampsia; systemic lupus erythematosus; in vitro fertilization

67. The criteria for pre-eclampsia include

- New onset elevated BP (SBP >140 mm Hg or DBP > 90 mm Hg on two occasions at least 4 hours apart or > 160/110 mm Hg) after 20 weeks of gestation and
- Proteinuria or
- New onset thrombocytopenia, renal insufficiency, impaired liver function, pulmonary edema, or cerebral/visual symptoms

68. What is first line therapy for endometriosis?

Combination oral contraceptives

69. Late in a pregnancy, a woman develops severe pruritus associated with papules and plaques. What is the likely diagnosis?

Pruritic urticarial papules and plaques of pregnancy (PUPPP)

70. When treating *Chlamydia,* how long should a patient wait before engaging in intercourse?

7 days

71. What is a vasa previa?

Vasa previa is when blood vessels within the placenta or the umbilical cord are trapped between the fetus and the birth canal, increasing risk of hemorrhage due to a blood vessel injury when the fetal membranes rupture or during labor and delivery.

72. What factors increase the risk for placental abruption?

Prior abruption (strongest risk factor)
Cocaine and other drug abuse
Abdominal trauma
Eclampsia
Preeclampsia or chronic HTN
Smoking during pregnancy
Increased maternal age
Increased parity

73. What is the worrisome cause of severe abdominal pain and vaginal bleeding in the third trimester

Placental abruption until proven otherwise

74. What is the likely diagnosis of a patient that has a frothy vaginal discharge with a pH >4.5? On exam she has a "strawberry cervix."

Trichomonas vaginalis

75. What is the treatment of choice *Trichomonas vaginalis*?

Oral metronidazole; the partner should also be treated.

76. Postmenopausal endometrial thickness greater than what measurement would suggest the possibility of endometrial hyperplasia or carcinoma?

5 mm

---

77. Folic acid is used to prevent what birth defect?

Neural tube defects; patients planning a pregnancy should take a daily supplement of 0.4–0.8 mg at least 1 month prior to conception. Women with a prior history of a pregnancy affected by a neural tube defect should take 4 mg/day.

---

78. A woman has cystic swelling lateral to the vaginal opening; you diagnose an infected Bartholin gland cyst. What is the treatment?

If infected, mainstay treatment is incision and drainage (I&D) with insertion of Word catheter. Marsupialization is more invasive and done in the Operating Room (OR) if it fails to resolve with one or two placements of Word catheter. If Bartholin cyst is asymptomatic, no treatment is necessary.

---

79. What is a missed abortion?

Missed abortion is defined as a dead fetus or embryo without passage of tissue, with a closed cervix.

---

80. What is a blighted ovum?

Blighted ovum is defined as a failure of the embryo to develop despite the presence of a gestational sac and placental tissue.

---

81. During pregnancy, what is the most common cause of jaundice?

Viral hepatitis

---

82. About 3 months following an uncomplicated delivery, a woman develops symptoms of anxiety, unexplained weight loss, and a rapid heart rate. A few months later, she develops fatigue, dry skin, and constipation. What is the likely diagnosis?

Postpartum thyroiditis; it develops following an uncomplicated delivery in two phases. The inflammation of the first phase induces symptoms of hyperthyroidism including anxiety, weight loss, tachycardia, and heat sensitivity; TSH will be suppressed. The second phase has symptoms of hypothyroidism, including fatigue, dry skin, cold sensitivity, and constipation; here, the TSH will be elevated. The condition is self-limiting within 18 months.

83. How is postpartum thyroiditis with an elevated TSH treated?

Thyroid replacement hormone for 6–12 months; at that time the medication can be stopped and TSH level rechecked 6 weeks later to determine if the hypothyroid condition has resolved.

84. A few days after an uncomplicated delivery, the mother develops irritability, bouts of crying, and anxiety. What is the likely diagnosis?

Baby blues, which begin within 1–2 weeks after delivery and resolves with reassurance; the ability to care for self and baby is preserved.

85. What are the symptoms of postpartum depression?

Postpartum depression may begin within a week after delivery. It may last for months and involves extreme depression with loss of ability to care for self or child.

86. What are the dangers of maternal parvovirus B19 infection?

Maternal parvovirus B19 in the first trimester can lead to spontaneous abortion; if infection occurs late in pregnancy, it can cause destruction of fetal red blood cells leading to anemia, heart failure, and fetal hydrops.

87. How is gestational hypertension (HTN) defined?

New onset of HTN at ≥ 20 weeks gestation, in absence of proteinuria, and/or end organ dysfunction.
Systolic blood pressure (SBP) ≥ 140 mm Hg or diastolic blood pressure (DBP) ≥ 90 mm Hg on at least two separate readings during pregnancy

88. What converts pre-eclampsia to eclampsia?

The onset of seizures or coma in someone with pre-eclampsia

89. In what condition is screening for asymptomatic bacteriuria recommended?

Pregnant women should be screened for asymptomatic bacteriuria with a urine culture at 12–16 weeks' gestation. There is no data to support testing or treatment of asymptomatic men or nonpregnant women regardless of age or underlying condition.

Obstetrics and Gynecology

90. Postcoital contraception with an intrauterine device (IUD) is effective if inserted within how many days?

Within 5 days

91. How should a newborn be treated if the mother is hepatitis B surface antigen positive?

Hepatitis B immunoglobulin (HBIG) and the first injection of the hepatitis B vaccination series should be administered within 12 hours of birth.

92. Women who develop cholestasis of pregnancy are at higher risk for postpartum cholestasis if exposed to what medication class?

Oral contraceptives can induce steroid-induced cholestasis.

93. What is the first-line treatment for primary dysmenorrhea?

NSAIDs (i.e., naproxen)

94. What intervention can be done to treat endometriosis if first-line therapies do not control symptoms?

For endometriosis not responsive to cyclic oral contraceptives, the patient may be tried on continuous contraception for 3–6 months or if there is chronic, noncyclic pelvic pain, placement of Levonorgestrel intrauterine device (IUD) will help.

95. What are the first-line of therapies for endometriosis?

NSAIDs for the pain and combined oral contraceptives

96. In a patient with known antiphospholipid antibody syndrome, what outcomes during pregnancy are increased?

Thromboembolism, recurrent fetal loss, thrombocytopenia

97. Chronic-glucocorticoids administered during pregnancy can result in

Increased risk of cleft palate, gestational diabetes, pregnancy-induced HTN, premature rupture of membranes, fetal growth restriction, infection, osteoporosis

98. In patients with what cancer is cancer antigen (CA) 125 used as a marker for treatment?

Ovarian cancer; there is strong evidence demonstrating no benefit and increased harm when used for screening and should NOT be used for this purpose.

99. Where should a fetal monitor be placed when a baby presents with mentum anterior?

The chin

100. When evaluating a woman for polycystic ovarian syndrome (PCOS), what LH:FSH ratio is consistent with the syndrome?

Greater than 2.5:1

101. What conditions decrease alfa fetoprotein?

Gestational age older than expected, trisomy (Down syndrome), hydatidiform mole, fetal demise, increased maternal weight

102. How is a screening done for gestational diabetes?

100 g 3-hour oral glucose tolerance test OR 75 g 2-hour oral glucose tolerance test

103. What is the best test for the detection of symptomatic renal stones in a pregnant female?

Ultrasound; there is no radiation exposure as with CT scans.

104. For what cancer is CA 27.29 used as a marker?

Breast cancer

Obstetrics and Gynecology

105. What conditions increase alfa fetoprotein?

Gestational age younger than expected, Neural tube defects: spina bifida, anencephaly, congenital skin defects, GI disorders (obstruction, liver disease, cloacal exstrophy), renal diseases (urinary obstruction, polycystic kidney disease), osteogenesis imperfecta, low birth weight, oligohydramnios, multiple gestations, decreased maternal weight

---

106. What are the initial treatments for PCOS?

Use of metformin, weight loss by way of reduced carbohydrate intake, exercise, and oral contraceptives

---

107. When a fetus has Down syndrome, what is the effect on the serum hCG level?

Serum hCG is about twice as high compared to an unaffected fetus.

---

108. When a pregnant female is found to have an elevated alfa fetoprotein level, what diagnostic test should be done next?

Obstetrical ultrasound

---

109. When during pregnancy should screening for gestational diabetes be done?

24–28 weeks' gestation

---

110. Patients with PCOS who want to get pregnant should be treated with what drug?

Clomiphene

---

111. How long after birth does physiologic jaundice and bilirubin peak?

Days 3–4

112. When gestational tropho-blastic disease (hydatid-iform mole) is suspected, what serum level should be obtained?

β-hCG (β-subunit of human chorionic gonadotropin)

113. How should women with hepatitis C wishing to breastfeed be counseled?

Breast milk and breastfeeding does not transmit HCV; mothers with hepatitis C can breastfeed. However, if nipples are cracked or bleeding, they should temporarily stop breastfeeding.

114. What nonhormonal medications are options for treating menopausal vasomotor instability?

Paroxetine (Paxil) and venlafaxine (Effexor); gabapentin (Neurontin) may also be used.

115. Patients who are PPD converters during pregnancy without active disease should receive what therapy?

INH plus pyridoxine (vitamin B_6)

116. Vacuum extraction may be attempted how many times?

Three

117. In vacuum extraction, where should the cup be placed?

The cup should be placed over the sagittal suture and about 3 cm in front of the posterior fontanel.

118. What is the risk of repairing episiotomies with skin sutures?

Skin sutures increase the incidence of perineal pain at 3 months after delivery.

119. What dose of folic acid is recommended for women who have previously given birth to children with neural tube defects?

4 mg daily

120. What dose of folic acid is recommended for women with no risk factors for neural tube defects?	400 µg daily
121. In pregnant women with history of prior DVT, what drug should be given to lower the risk of a DVT recurring during subsequent pregnancies?	Low molecular weight heparin (warfarin is teratogenic).
122. Pruritus gravidarum associated with severe pruritus in the third trimester is due to	Intrahepatic cholestasis
123. What is a darkening of the skin of the face during pregnancy and with oral contraceptive use called?	Melasma
124. True or false: acetaminophen is considered safe in all trimesters of pregnancy.	True
125. What should you check in a pregnant woman with severe generalized pruritus but no obvious dermatosis?	Bile acid and LFTs for intrahepatic cholestasis of pregnancy
126. True or false: NSAIDs are considered safe in all trimesters of pregnancy.	False: although commonly used, they may cause increased risks of miscarriage and malformations early in the pregnancy and exposure after 30 weeks' gestation is associated with an increased risk of premature closure of the fetal ductus arteriosus and oligohydramnios.

127. True or false: H2 antagonists and proton pump inhibitors are considered safe in all trimesters of pregnancy.

True, they are believed safe, but are only to be dosed on a daily basis if antacids or prn use is ineffective.

128. For women in preterm labor, what agents can be used as tocolytics?

Terbutaline, magnesium sulfate, and nifedipine

129. On screening ultrasound, the finding of an increased nuchal translucency seen at 10–14 weeks is consistent with what diagnosis?

Down syndrome

130. Use of estrogen without progesterone can increase the risk of what condition?

Endometrial hyperplasia and endometrial cancer

131. What is infarction of the pituitary gland during labor and delivery called?

Sheehan syndrome symptoms include inability to lactate, amenorrhea, and other symptoms of loss of pituitary function

132. What is a common presentation of Sheehan syndrome?

Difficulty with breastfeeding after delivery

133. Which partner should be evaluated first in an infertility evaluation?

Male (sperm analysis); the female evaluation is more extensive and expensive.

134. How does basal body temperature change during ovulation?

It increases from 0.58°F to 1.08°F.

Obstetrics and Gynecology

135. How should women be counseled to sleep after 20 weeks' gestation?	Pregnant women should sleep on their left side; sleeping on their back allows the enlarged uterus to possibly compress the great vessels leading to compromised blood flow to the uterus.
136. What is the first test that should be done in women of childbearing age who present with abnormal uterine bleeding?	Serum hCG levels to check for pregnancy
137. During labor a woman develops severe abdominal pain and/or has a tender uterus. What diagnosis should be ruled out?	Placental abruption
138. What is the most common cause of excessive bleeding in the immediate postpartum period?	Uterine atony
139. How is uterine atony treated following delivery?	Vigorous fundal massage and intravenous oxytocin
140. What is the drug of choice for eclamptic seizures?	Magnesium sulfate
141. What maneuver should be done first for the treatment of shoulder dystocia?	McRoberts maneuver, sharp hyperflexion of the mother's thighs toward the mother's abdomen
142. What concerns are raised with repetitive variable decelerations found on fetal heart tracings?	Umbilical cord compression

143. Repetitive late decelerations noted on fetal heart tracings during labor suggest what condition? — Uteroplacental insufficiency

144. How many additional calories do pregnant women need per day? — 300 calories

145. What is the leading cause of nonobstetrical death in pregnant women? — Trauma; Motor vehicle accidents (MVAs) are the most common cause, followed by assault.

146. How is preterm labor defined? — Traditionally, preterm labor is defined as <37 weeks and term labor between 38 and 42 weeks.

147. What is early term labor? — Early term labor is between 37 weeks 0 days and 38 weeks 6 days.

148. How is full-term labor defined? — Full term labor is between 39 weeks 0 days and 40 weeks 6 days.

149. How is late-term labor defined? — Late term labor is between 41 weeks 0 days and 41 weeks 6 days.

150. How is post-term labor defined? — Post term labor is between 42 weeks 0 days and beyond.

151. Which HPV subtypes are most commonly associated with cervical cancer? — Types 16 and 18

152. What bacteria is the most common cause of neonatal sepsis in the United States? — Group B *Streptococcus*

153.	How does breast conservation surgery in women with breast cancer affect their body image?	Improved body image Higher satisfaction with treatment No greater fear of recurrence compared with women treated with mastectomy
154.	What part of a woman's menstrual cycle is the ideal time to perform a clinical breast examination in premenopausal women?	1 week after menses, when breasts are least swollen and tender
155.	What is the most common presentation of ectopic pregnancy?	Abdominal pain and spotting in the first 6–8 weeks after the last menstrual period is commonly associated with ectopic pregnancy.
156.	When spotting occurs in the first trimester, what laboratory test is useful in distinguishing a viable pregnancy from an ectopic pregnancy?	A β-hCG level that doubles in 48 hours is more likely to be a viable pregnancy. Correlate with findings of intra uterine pregnancy (IUP) on transvaginal ultrasound.
157.	To estimate gestational age during the first trimester, what ultrasound-based measurement is used?	During ultrasound in the first trimester, the crown-rump length best predicts gestational age.
158.	At how many weeks can an external version be attempted?	36 weeks' gestation
159.	If using magnesium sulfate for eclampsia, what life-threatening side effect may occur?	Respiratory depression can be induced by magnesium sulfate.
160.	What is the treatment regimen for uncomplicated gonococcal infections?	The recommended regimen is a single dose ceftriaxone IM and single dose azithromycin oral dose.

161. During pregnancy and in all patients, what is the drug of choice for treating of syphilis?

Penicillin G

162. In preterm labor, what medication may be given prior to delivery to reduce mortality and morbidity (respiratory distress syndrome and intraventricular hemorrhage)?

Corticosteroids

163. How does the lecithin-sphingomyelin (L/S) ratio and phosphatidylglycerol (PG) in preterm labor to determine lung maturity in the fetus?

Respiratory distress syndrome (RDS) is rare if the L/S ratio is > 2 and PG is present. If the L/S ratio is < 2 but PG is present, RDS develops in < 5% of infants.

164. What percent of recognized pregnancies end in miscarriage?

Approximately 15%

165. What drug is used to terminate an ectopic pregnancy? What must you rule out prior to starting medical treatment?

Methotrexate (MTX)
Must rule out viable intrauterine pregnancy

166. In a pregnant patient with mild persistent asthma, what medication should be used to prevent asthma exacerbations?

Inhaled corticosteroids

167. A vaginal discharge with a pH <4.5 implies what common infection?

Candida vulvovaginitis

168. What are the effective and safe methods to treat pregnancy-induced nausea?

Acupressure, ginger, pyridoxine (vitamin B$_6$)

169. What are the treatment options for women under 35 at low risk for uterine cancer with anovulatory bleeding?

Combination oral contraceptives (ethinyl estradiol $\leq$ 35 µg) or progesterone (Provera) 10 mg/day for days 10–14 days/month.

170. Define premenstrual dysphoric disorder.

Premenstrual dysphoric disorder (PMDD) is a severe form of PMS characterized by severe recurrent depressive and anxiety symptoms, with premenstrual (luteal phase) onset, which remits a few days after the start of menses.

171. Define advanced maternal age.

Traditionally at least 35 years of age or estimated delivery date older than age 35

172. What vaccines should not be given during pregnancy?

Measles, mumps, and rubella (MMR)
Varicella

1. Use of clozapine is associated with what blood abnormality?

Agranulocytosis; patients on clozapine should have serial CBCs.

2. What condition is associated with recurrent episodes of quickly eating large quantities of food, often to the point of discomfort, a loss of control during the eating, shame or guilt afterward, and not purging, or abusing laxatives called?

Binge eating disorder

3. For mania, what antiseizure medication can be used?

Valproate

4. In patients with anorexia nervosa, what cardiac related finding is induced?

Bradycardia

5. What psychiatric medications can cause serotonin syndrome?

Selective serotonin reuptake inhibitors (SSRIs), serotonin-norepinephrine reuptake inhibitors (SNRIs), monoamine oxidase inhibitors (MAOIs), bupropion, tricyclic antidepressants (TCAs), lithium, herbal supplements (including St. John's Wort), and some illicit drugs

6. How is binge eating disorder different from anorexia nervosa?

Binge eating disorder is similar to an addiction, where self-image is intact but control over eating is not. Anorexia is considered distortion of self-image. Cognitive behavioral therapy (CBT) and psychotherapy are used for both, although binge eating disorder may respond to some medications (topiramate, stimulants).

7. What does the psychiatric axis 1 define?	Axis 1: High-level diagnosis; acute symptoms that need treatment (e.g., major depressive episode, schizophrenic episode, panic attack)
8. What is the most common eating disorder in the United States?	Binge eating disorder
9. What does the psychiatric Axis 2 define?	Axis 2: Personality disorders A: Paranoid, schizoid, schizotypal B: Antisocial, borderline, histrionic, narcissistic C: Avoidant, dependent, obsessive, compulsive
10. For patients on SSRIs who develop serotonin syndrome, what medications can be used to treat the symptoms?	Benzodiazepines and cyproheptadine (Periactin)
11. What does the Psychiatric Axis 3 define?	Axis 3: Medical diagnosis (e.g., diabetes, asthma, etc.)
12. What does the Psychiatric Axis 4 define?	Axis 4: Recent psychosocial stressors
13. What does the Psychiatric Axis 5 define?	Axis 5: Global assessment of functioning (GAF) scaled 0–100 (where 100 is ideal) on ability to function in daily life
14. A 22-year-old woman presents with a body mass index (BMI) of < 15 and has secondary amenorrhea for 3 months; urine hCG is negative. What is the likely cause of her amenorrhea?	Patients with anorexia nervosa can induce secondary amenorrhea (loss of menstrual bleeding); patients with bulimia do not routinely develop amenorrhea.

Psychiatry

15. What are the components of the Patient Health Questionnaire 9 (PHQ-9)?

In the last 2 weeks, how often have you felt
1. Sleep (trouble falling or staying asleep, or sleeping too much)
2. Interest (little interest or pleasure)
3. Guilt (feeling badly about yourself; let others down)
4. Energy (tired, little energy)
5. Concentration (trouble watching TV or reading)
6. Appetite changes (poor appetite or overeating)
7. Psychomotor changes (lethargic, moving slowly, or manic)
8. Suicidal/Homicidal thoughts (better off dead or gone)
9. Depressed feeling (hopeless)

16. What are the components of a gambling disorder?

Gambling disorder is persistent and recurrent maladaptive gambling behavior that disrupts personal, family, and/or vocational pursuits. It has high rates of comorbidity with other mental disorders (substance use, depression, anxiety, and personality disorders).

17. What the classic behaviors of someone with histrionic personality disorder?

Histrionic personality disorder is often expressed as excessive emotions and attention seeking. People with this disorder have attractive, flamboyant personalities.

18. What is dysthymia?

A chronic depressive disorder (lasting more than 2 years) associated with an early and insidious onset (i.e., in childhood, adolescence, or early adulthood)

19. How does depression differ from dysthymia?

Depression requires a majority of the PHQ 9 responses to be positive, has a more acute onset, and when treated, depression goes into remission. Dysthymia requires a minority of PHQ 9 positive responses, and rarely goes into remission.

Psychiatry

20. A 22-year-old veteran is seen in follow-up from an Emergency Department visit for a boxer's fracture of his hand; he seems distant and admits to frequently getting into fights. What condition should he be evaluated for?

Posttraumatic stress disorder (PTSD); this is an anxiety disorder defined as a reaction that can occur after exposure to an extreme traumatic event involving death, threat of death, serious physical injury, or a threat to physical integrity. This reaction has three cardinal characteristics: reexperiencing the trauma, avoidance of anything related to the traumatic event and/or numbing of general responsiveness, and an increased arousal.

21. What are the common traits of somatization disorder?

Onset before 30 years of age
Rarely affects males
Physical and/or sexual abuse
Multiple symptoms affecting multiple organ systems
Not logical history given, jumping to multiple symptoms during interview
Anxious and depressed
Suicide attempts are common.

22. What are the common behaviors of someone with borderline personality disorder?

Impulsivity
Unstable relationships
Difficulty regulating behavior
Unstable mood
Self-damaging acts
Boredom, feelings of emptiness, depression
Paranoia
Extreme dependency
Alternating idealization and devaluation of the physician

23. What characteristics and populations are at high risk for suicide?

Age over 45
Male gender
Caucasian race
Living alone
Poor health

24. What sexual side effect is associated with trazodone?

Priapism

25. What sexual side effects are associated with SSRIs?

Decreased libido
Delayed ejaculation
Anorgasmia

26. What are the treatments of choice for posttraumatic stress disorder?

CBT, relaxation techniques including meditation and when medication is needed, SSRIs.

27. What metabolic disorder is associated atypical antipsychotic medications?

Type 2 diabetes mellitus

28. What condition is associated with symptoms of illness in a child that are exaggerated, fabricated, or induced by a caretaker when there is usually no underlying health disorder in the child?

Munchausen syndrome by proxy or factitious disorder by proxy; results in harm to the child victim through repeated interactions with the medical care system, including unnecessary tests, medications, and surgeries.

29. For panic disorder, what medication class is the treatment of choice?

SSRIs

30. For obsessive-compulsive disorder, what class of drugs should be used as first line of treatment?

SSRIs

31. For bipolar disease, what agents are commonly used as first line of treatment?

Lithium, antiseizure medication, atypical antipsychotics

32. What endocrinologic disorder can lithium induce?

Hypothyroidism; in women up to 15% will develop hypothyroidism; in men ~5%

Psychiatry

33. What are the common criteria to commit someone for mental illness against his/her will?

Commitment criteria: (1) Individual is mentally ill (many states exclude mental retardation, antisocial behavior, medical illness, and substance abuse); (2) High likelihood of serious harm (substantial risk of physical harm to self OR substantial risk of physical harm to other persons OR "Gravely disabled": inability to care for basic needs, including food, clothing, shelter, medical care, and safety; (3) No less-restrictive alternative to hospitalization would attenuate risk. There are two stages of commitment: (a) Emergency detention and admission (sometimes called emergency hold)—an emergency admission with minimum of legal process, usually 72 hr and (b) Longer-term commitment—requires judicial approval of continued confinement in an adversarial proceeding where patient may have legal representation.

34. How do you determine the difference between delirium and dementia?

To determine the difference, look at the onset of symptoms. Delirium develops acutely with rapid deterioration over hours to days whereas dementia develops over months to years.

35. In treating mania, what mood stabilizer drugs are commonly used?

Lithium carbonate
Valproic acid
Carbamazepine
Lamotrigine

36. Describe the signs and symptoms associated with mania.

Increased psychomotor activity
Euphoria
Impaired judgment
Impulsivity
Grandiose ideas
Irritability

37. As a child with attention deficit hyperactivity disorder ages, what symptoms may persist into adulthood?

Inattention
Hyperactivity and impulsivity tend to decrease with advancing age.

38. What is the common side effect of electroconvulsive therapy (ECT) on mental status?

Reversible short-term memory loss

39. What are the six stages of change?

- Precontemplation
- Contemplation
- Determination
- Action
- Maintenance
- Termination

40. What psychiatric diagnosis is associated with thought disorders such as hallucinations, delusions, and loose associations, disorganized speech, catatonic behavior, and apathy or flat affect resulting in social/occupational impairment?

Schizophrenia

41. What test is helpful in detecting polypharmacy?

Urine toxicology screen

42. Long-term use of which anticonvulsive agent is associated with osteoporosis?

Phenytoin

43. What is the risk when an SSRI is used in the treatment of bipolar disorder?

SSRIs may induce mania in patients with bipolar disorder.

44. Define hypochondriasis.

Hypochondriasis is a preoccupation with bodily functions and fears of acquiring a serious disease.

Psychiatry

45. Define the clinical signs and symptoms of a conversion disorder.

Conversion disorder is a set of physical symptoms related to a psychological conflict that are unconsciously converted to a neurologic disorder (lack of coordination or balance, weakness, paralysis, loss of sensation, simulated convulsions, or loss of major senses).

46. What is the likely diagnosis in a patient with daily excessive anxiety and worry that has continued for more than 6 months?

Generalized anxiety disorder

47. In diagnosing a primary mood disorder, what is the most important predisposing factor?

Family history

48. Which antidepressant medication can be used in smoking cessation and is associated with seizures but does not cause significant sexual dysfunction?

Bupropion (Wellbutrin)

49. What class of antidepressant drugs can induce a hypertensive crisis if mixed with tyramine-containing products such as aged cheese?

MAOIs.

50. In the evaluation of primary erectile dysfunction (ED), what is the most common cause?

Psychogenic causes (guilt, fear, depression, anxiety) can be distinguished from a physiologic cause as people with psychogenic ED continue to get nocturnal and morning erections, while those with physiologic ED do not.

51. What nonpharmaco-logic treatment can be used for circadian sleep disorders? — Bright light therapy

52. What condition is characterized by two or more identities or personalities? — Dissociative identity disorder

53. Which SSRI is most likely to induce loose stools? — Sertraline (Zoloft)

54. Which antidepressant is useful in the treatment of weight loss in the elderly? — Mirtazapine (Remeron)

55. Which antidepressive medication can induce an elevation in diastolic blood pressure? — Venlafaxine (Effexor)

56. What class of medication is likely to causing yawn-ing as a side effect? — SSRIs

57. Which antidepressant medications are highly sedative and can be used to treat insomnia? — Trazodone, doxepin, most TCAs (amitriptyline)

58. What is the first mode of treatment for bulimia? — Cognitive behavioral therapy

59. What drugs are approved for lowering the risk of alcohol abuse relapse? — Naltrexone, acamprosate (Campral), topiramate

Psychiatry

60. What drugs are used to lower the risk of seizures and delirium in alcohol withdrawal?

Long-acting benzodiazepines (BZDs) (diazepam, chlordiazepoxide) are more effective at preventing breakthrough seizures and delirium management.

61. In the United States, what medication is approved for the treatment of bulimia?

Fluoxetine (Prozac)

62. What neurotransmitter is affected by the use of acamprosate (Campral)?

γ-Aminobutyric acid (GABA)

63. What type of interpersonal therapy is recommended in obsessive compulsive disorder?

Cognitive behavioral therapy

64. What medications can be used for the treatment of chronic opioid dependence?

Methadone, Suboxone (buprenorphine/naloxone)

65. Chronic use of methadone maintenance therapy decreases the risk of what other diseases?

HIV, hepatitis B and C

66. Does the use of β blockers increase the risk of depression?

There is no data that supports a significant increased risk of reported depressive symptoms when taking β blockers.

67. What are the five stages of sleep?

Stages 1, 2, 3, 4, and rapid eye movement (REM) sleep. They cycle from stage 1 to REM sleep, and then repeat.
Approximately 50% of sleep is in stage 2, 20% in REM sleep, and the rest in the other stages.

68. In which stage of sleep does dreaming occur?

REM sleep

Psychiatry

69. What happens to a patient's REM sleep as they age?

REM sleep does not change, but, there are significant decreases in stage 3 and 4 sleep.

70. On an EEG, how is wakefulness characterized?

Alpha Waves

71. In patients on lithium for bipolar disorder, what blood testing should be done on a regular basis?

Renal and thyroid functions

72. What is the goal of cognitive therapy?

To help the patient change a thought that leads to a change of mood, behavior, or reaction

73. What side effect is most common with St. John's wort?

Transient photosensitivity rash

74. In a patient with anorexia nervosa, what clinical findings are common?

Bradycardia, low blood pressure, pubertal delay, loss of tooth enamel

75. At a local middle school, an outbreak of nonspecific symptoms (headache, dizziness, lightheadedness, abdominal discomfort, chest discomfort, and inability to concentrate) occurs but no identifiable source is found. What is the term for this psychosomatic situation?

Mass psychogenic illness

76. What drug is used to prevent alcohol withdrawal in a patient with cirrhosis?

Short-acting benzodiazepine such as lorazepam (Ativan)

Psychiatry

77. What neurotransmitter is altered by alcohol consumption?	γ-Aminobutyric acid (GABA)
78. What are the clinical characteristics of baby blues?	Baby blues consist of mild depressive symptoms, crying without a cause, anxiety, irritability, and fatigue that can start within a few days of delivery and usually resolve within 10–14 days of birth.
79. Patients use SAMe (adenosylmethionine) as it is believed to alter what neurotransmitter?	Serotonin
80. If a patient on an SSRI or SNRI develops a decreased libido, what antidepressant medications can be used because they have little effect on libido?	Bupropion (Wellbutrin)
81. What condition is hoped to be prevented by taking ginko biloba?	Dementia
82. What conditions may be improved by the use of valerian root?	Insomnia and anxiety
83. What medication can induce a paradoxical reaction in patients with mental retardation?	Benzodiazepines
84. What is the worrisome side effect associated ginkgo biloba?	Bleeding complications
85. Kava has been used by eastern cultures to treat what condition?	Anxiety

86. What herb used for depression may reduce the effectiveness of oral contraceptives?

St. John's wort

87. What is the development of emotional or physical maladaptive symptoms that occur within 3 months following an identifiable stressor called?

Adjustment disorder

88. What older class of antidepressant medications can precipitate hypotension and arrhythmias?

TCAs

89. What antiepileptic drug is commonly used to treat chronic neuropathic pain?

Gabapentin (Neurontin).

90. What antiseizure medication is associated with rare but potentially life-threatening rashes?

Lamotrigine (Lamictal)

91. What method is used by males for suicide *completion*?

Gunshot (firearms)

92. What method of suicide is most commonly used by females?

Drug overdose

93. What cardiac condition abnormality does haloperidol potentially induce?

Prolongation of the Q–T interval

94. Who is most commonly the abuser in elder abuse?

A relative (usually the spouse)

Psychiatry

95. What is the primary treatment for seasonal affective disorder?	Light therapy for 30 min/day
96. Smoking affects what gynecological conditions?	Infertility, spontaneous abortion, ectopic pregnancy, and premature menopause
97. What are persistent thoughts, ideas, and images that invade conscious awareness called?	Obsessions
98. What term is used for urges or impulses for repetitive intentional behavior performed in a stereotyped manner?	Compulsions
99. What risk factors are associated with suicide?	Prior history of admission to a psychiatric facility Other risk factors include living in an urban area, being unemployed, single, and poor.
100. What metabolic condition does bulimia induce?	Metabolic alkalosis
101. Which TCA has the potential to induce the most anticholinergic properties (dry mouth, blurred vision, constipation, and urinary retention)?	Amitriptyline
102. Venlafaxine alters which neurotransmitters?	Serotonin and norepinephrine

103. Sleep disturbance, decreased interest or pleasure, feelings of worthlessness or guilt, fatigue, difficulty with concentration, altered appetite, weight change, psychomotor agitation or depression, and active suicidal thoughts that exist for at least 2 weeks are consistent with what diagnosis?

Depression

104. When anorexia is successfully treated, in what percent of women does menstruation usually resume?

90%

105. What condition is likely when a patient taking haloperidol develops a high fever, tachycardia, tachypnea, diaphoresis, and mental status changes?

Neuroleptic malignant syndrome

106. What eye-related condition has been associated with quetiapine (Seroquel) use?

Cataract formation
Screening for cataracts is recommended at the initiation of therapy and at 6-month intervals thereafter.

107. Disulfiram (Antabuse) can continue to react with alcohol for how many days after the drug is discontinued?

Up to 14 days

108. How soon after starting an antidepressant should the patient be followed up?

2–3 weeks

Psychiatry

109. What condition would upper dental erosions in a 22-year-old female college student suggest?

Bulimia nervosa

110. A patient presents with mildly depressed mood, fatigue, low self-esteem, difficulty with concentration, and persistent hopelessness for at least 2 years. What is the likely diagnosis?

Dysthymia

111. What condition involves episodes of dysthymia followed by episodes of mild mania?

Cyclothymia

112. What disorder is likely if a female patient has issues of impulsivity, victimization, dependency, limited insight, and alternating episodes of idolization and disgust with her physician?

Borderline personality disorder

113. What is the likely diagnosis for someone with a pattern of one or more somatic symptoms recurring or persisting for > 6 months that are distressing or result in significant disruption of daily life, with no identifiable cause, is not being faked, and is true suffering by the patient?

Somatization disorder

Psychiatry

114. What antianxiety medication does not induce dependence or cause abuse, cause drowsiness, or other functional limitations and is safe for senior citizens?

Buspirone (Buspar)

115. Abrupt cessation of what class of psychiatric medication can cause headaches, anxiety, diarrhea, dizziness, fatigue, insomnia, and visual disturbances?

SSRIs

116. What is the neurosis in which the patient fakes signs or symptoms without tangible personal benefit other than to experience the sick role, is more common in men, and a chronic childhood illness?

Munchausen syndrome

117. What common past medical/social history is found in a patient with Munchausen syndrome?

Parental emotional or physical abuse

118. How does Munchausen syndrome differ from factitious disorder?

Factitious disorder patients tend to simulate only one disease and they do this during times of major psychosocial stress. They do not doctor shop (as those with Munchausen syndrome) and they usually can be treated successfully.

119. What treatment is commonly used for Munchausen disorder?

Confronting the patient with the diagnosis without suggesting guilt or reproach

Psychiatry

120. How is somatization disorder treated?	Treatment consists of arranging a regular visit on an agreed-upon interval to help limit emergency department (ED) exposure and unnecessary testing and a long-term physician relationship that offers reassurance and symptomatic relief when necessary but discourages unnecessary diagnostic or therapeutic procedures. Medications and psychotherapy may be beneficial.
121. What is the most common cause of death in adults below age 50 years?	Prescription drug accidental overdose (opioids are the class with the greatest risk)
122. In motivational interviewing, what two aspects should a practitioner assess with a patient?	Patient's level of importance about the issues and his or her confidence about achieving it
123. What is the likely diagnosis when a patient describes excessive/irrational fear and avoidance of situations that may be difficult to escape, including fear of crowds, enclosed spaces (e.g., elevators, automobiles, or airplanes), or simply being alone (at home or away from home) and is often associated with panic disorder?	Agoraphobia
124. How is agoraphobia treated?	Agoraphobia is treated by exposure therapy where the patient confronts and remains within the environment they fear until anxiety resolves (this is called habituation).

Psychiatry

125. In the general adult population, what are the most common anxiety disorders?

Phobias (fear of snakes, dark, flying, heights, needles, etc.) present in up to 7% of individuals.

126. How long must buspirone be taken to begin to show anxiolytic effects?

About 2 weeks

127. What is the condition associated with a stressful event inducing a memory lapse that can range from a few minutes to years?

Dissociative amnesia

128. What is the term when a patient has the inability to form new memories after an event?

Antegrade amnesia

129. What condition is characterized by the assumption of a new name and identity following a major stressful event (i.e., major accidents, and natural disasters)?

Dissociative fugue

130. What is the condition called when previously stored memories are unavailable?

Retrograde amnesia, most often temporary

131. In geriatric depression, how common is suicide among depressed men?

Suicide rates are highest for males aged > 75 years (rate 38.5/100,000).

Psychiatry

132. What conditions are included on the differential diagnosis for senior citizens with new onset depression?	Hypothyroidism, vitamin B_{12} deficiency, liver or renal failure, cancers, stroke, new onset dementia, some medications
133. What diagnosis has the highest risk for suicide?	Dissociative identity disorder (multiple personality disorder)
134. What is the clinical state when a patient feels removed from himself or herself, and detached from his or her physical and mental processes?	Depersonalization
135. Overdose of TCAs may cause what fatal condition?	Cardiac arrhythmia
136. At higher dosages, what SSRI is associated with weight loss and is effective for binge eating disorder?	Fluoxetine (Prozac)
137. How does trazodone effect blood pressure?	Trazodone is a α_1-noradrenergic antagonist and is associated with postural hypotension.
138. Because of its adverse effects, which patients should not be prescribed bupropion?	Patients with seizure disorders
139. In patients with severe depression refractory to medication, what intervention may be considered?	Electroconvulsive therapy

140. What clinical condition can chronic lithium use induce?

Hypothyroidism
This can be ruled out by obtaining a thyroid stimulating hormone (TSH) level.

141. Which class of antihypertensives can induce lithium toxicity in patients using lithium for bipolar disorder?

Diuretics

142. Why should lithium not be used in women who may become pregnant?

Lithium use in the first trimester may induce Ebstein anomaly, a cardiac defect.

143. Carbamazepine and divalproex use in the first trimester are associated with what birth defect?

Neural tube defects

144. What personality disorder is associated with distrust of others' motives resulting in avoidance of intimate relationships, grudges, and the sense that they are being exploited by others?

Paranoid personality disorder

145. What personality disorder is most commonly seen by healthcare providers?

Borderline personality disorder

146. What personality disorder is associated with grandiosity, exaggerated sense of superiority, and often seen in individuals who are high achievers?

Narcissistic personality disorder

Psychiatry

147. A person who demonstrates a habitual pattern of passive resistance to expected work requirements, expresses opposition, and has negative attitudes in response to requirements for normal performance is what personality type?	Passive aggressive personality
148. What childhood exposure can result in chronic hypoactive sexual desire?	Abuse or traumatic events in childhood
149. A side effect of what class of medication can be used to treat premature ejaculation?	SSRIs
150. What is the term for patients who obtain sexual satisfaction by observing unsuspecting persons who are naked, disrobing, or engaging in sexual activity?	Voyeurs
151. What factor has the greatest impact on the prognosis for patients with schizophrenia?	Adherence to prescribed psychoactive medications
152. Antipsychotic medication can induce what condition which presents with involuntary movement such as puckering of the lips and tongue and/or writhing of the arms or legs?	Tardive dyskinesia

153. What potentially fatal adverse event may result from the use of antipsychotic medication associated with rigidity, fever, autonomic instability, and elevated creatinine phosphokinase?

Neuroleptic malignant syndrome

154. What vitamin can prevent the cerebellar degeneration seen in alcoholics?

B_1 (Thiamine)

155. For mild to moderate depression, what treatment is as effective as medication?

Cognitive behavioral therapy

156. What should be administered to unconscious patients before IV glucose?

Thiamine should be given IV to prevent Wernicke encephalopathy and Korsakoff psychosis.

157. What is included in the differential diagnosis of adult attention deficit disorder (ADD)?

Hearing impairment, thyroid dysfunction, sleep deprivation, sleep apnea, phenylketonuria, obsessive-compulsive disorder (OCD), lead toxicity, substance abuse

158. What is the single greatest risk factor of adult ADD?

Having attention deficit hyperactivity disorder (ADHD) symptoms before age 12 years

Psychiatry

159. What diagnosis is present in patients with pervasive subjective feelings of ugliness about one or more aspects of their appearance despite a normal or near-normal appearance?

Body dysmorphic disorder
DSM V criteria (all must be included):

■ Preoccupation with a perceived defect in appearance. If there is a minor physical anomaly, the concern is excessive.

■ At some point during the course of the disorder, the individual has performed repetitive behaviors or mental acts in response to the appearance concerns.

■ The preoccupation causes clinically significant distress or impairment in social, occupational, or other important areas of function.

■ The preoccupation is not accounted for by another mental disorder or meet criteria for an eating disorder.

160. What is the drug class of choice for body dysmorphic disorder?

SSRIs

161. What condition occurs in children when provoked by strong emotion to seem to stop breathing, become limp, and possibly become unresponsive, but are not having a seizure?

Breath holding attacks characterized by the following:

■ Emotionally provoked attacks in children 1–7 years; can progress from a strong emotion to breath holding to decreased sensorium and either limpness or stiffness, which can appear as seizure-like activity.

■ Disease essentials:
  • Provoked by anger, pain, or frustration
  • Association with altered respiratory effort
  • Results in decreased muscle tone
  • Can be classified as simple (brief, no loss of consciousness) or severe (prolonged, associated loss of consciousness)

162. What percent of teenagers experience cyberbullying?

Estimated to be at 15%, cyberbullying is behavior via electronic or digital media that communicates hostile or aggressive messages intended to harm or cause discomfort to others. Three-fourths of victims report knowing their bully implying that one-fourth of those bullied report NOT knowing their victim.

163. What is the likely diagnosis of a 27-year-old with history of recurrent depression episodes who now presents agitated, speech is pressured, has flight of ideas, and is having grandiose or paranoid thoughts?

Bipolar I (BP-I) is a mood disorder characterized by at least one manic or mixed episode, often alternating with episodes of major depression. Exam finds the following:

- General appearance: bright clothing, excessive makeup, disorganized or discombobulated, psychomotor agitation
- Speech: pressured, difficult to interrupt
- Mood/Affect: euphoria, irritability/expansive, labile
- Thought process: flight of ideas (streams of thought occur to patient at rapid rate), easily distracted
- Thought content: grandiosity, paranoia, hyperreligious
- Perceptual abnormalities: three-fourths of manic patients experience delusions, grandiose or paranoid
- Suicidal/homicidal ideation: Irritability or delusions may lead to aggression toward self or others; suicidal ideation is common with mixed episode.
- Insight/judgment: poor/impaired

164. How does bipolar II differ from bipolar I?

Bipolar II consists of at least one episode of major depression and at least one episode of hypomania, a milder form of mania. Bipolar I has mania, which includes flight of ideas and grandiose or paranoid thoughts.

Psychiatry

165. Hallucinations are sensory perceptions (auditory, olfactory, visual, tactile, gustatory) that occur without external stimulation of the relevant sensory organ but are experienced as a sensation through that organ. What medications can induce hallucinations?

- Anticholinergic agents
- Steroids
- Methylphenidate

166. What percent of homeless individuals suffer from chronic mental illness?

25%

167. What percent of homeless individuals are veterans?

8%

168. For patients with chronic insomnia, what are the components of good sleep hygiene?

Fixed wake-up times and bedtimes regardless of amount of sleep obtained (weekdays and weekends)
Go to bed only when sleepy.
Avoid naps.
Sleep in cool, dark, quiet environment.
No activities or stimuli in bedroom associated with anything but sleep or sex
30-minute wind-down time before sleep
If unable to sleep within 20 minutes, move to another environment and engage in quiet activity until sleepy.

169. What interventions should be first-line treatment for all patients with chronic insomnia?

Proper sleep hygiene and cognitive behavioral therapy

170. What percentage of patients with binge eating disorder and bulimia abuse laxatives?

Up to 70% of patients with binging/purging anorexia and bulimia nervosa abuse laxatives but rarely as the sole method of purging.

171. What is the most commonly used illicit substance in the United States?

Cannabis is the most widely used illicit psychoactive substance in the United States.

Approximately 42% of teens will have tried marijuana by the time they graduate from high school and approximately 30% of students report having used marijuana at college entry.

In the United States, 10% of those who ever used marijuana become daily users, and 20%–30% become weekly users.

172. What skin disorder is due to a habit or anxiety induced that results in skin lichenification (thickening)?

Lichen simplex chronicus is dermatitis resulting from chronic, repeated rubbing or scratching of the skin, resulting in thickening with accentuated lines ("lichenification"); the scratching may be secondary to habit or a conditioned response to anxiety.

173. What disorder causes at least two individuals to both hold the same delusional belief?

Shared delusional disorder occurs when a delusional belief held by one person (the "primary") becomes shared by one other (the "secondary") or several other people associated with that person. It is also known as shared psychotic disorder and folie a deux (if two people are involved).

Psychiatry

1. What medication is used following hip or knee surgery to prevent deep venous thrombosis (DVT)?

Low molecular weight heparin

2. A 60-year-old woman presents with sudden, painless unilateral vision loss; what is the most worrisome condition?

Central retinal artery occlusion; any sudden vision loss requires emergent evaluation by slit lamp.

3. What test is used to discern hip pain is from the sacroiliac joint vs the hip?

The FABER test (flexion, abduction, and external rotation of the hip) or Patrick test; pain in the sacroiliac area suggests sacroiliac joint dysfunction; pain may radiate to the groin.

4. What is the first intervention for snakebite?

Antivenom

5. An adult is hit in the face and has avulsed a tooth; how should it be handled?

Avoid touching tooth root; handle only by the crown; rinse with normal saline. If there is dirt or a large clot in the socket, perform gentle irrigation of the socket with normal saline. After implantation, have patient bite down on gauze while transporting to dentist. If unable to implant at scene, transport in Hanks solution, milk, or saline (not water) or the buccal sulcus if patient is alert and age-appropriate.

6. How many days after stopping aspirin will the risk of bleeding persist?

5 days; most groups recommend 7 days

7. For frostbite, what medications must be administered within the first 24 hours to lower amputation rates?

tPA to prevent thrombosis can lower the risk of amputation in frostbite.

---

8. In infants and children, what clinical finding is the first sign of shock?

Tachycardia

---

9. What ECG finding is suggestive of pericardial tamponade?

Electrical alternans (when consecutive QRS complexes alternate in height because of heart swinging in fluid) is seen in pericardial tamponade.

---

10. What feature differentiates superficial and deep frostbite?

Deep frostbite finds tissue mottled and pulseless after rewarming, with loss of sensation and rare hemorrhagic blisters. Superficial frostbite has erythema and edema with rewarming and blister formation.

---

11. When osteomyelitis is suspected, what is the test of choice?

Magnetic resonance imaging (MRI) is the most sensitive; leukocyte scans are also sensitive but not considered the first choice.

---

12. What are the three categories of the Glasgow Coma Scale and its interpretation?

Eye opening (1–4)
Verbal response (1–5)
Motor response (1–6)
Score 12 indicates severe head injury, score 8 suggests the need for intubation and ventilation, and score 6 suggests the need for intracranial pressure monitoring.

---

13. A young woman develops a cystic lesion over the posterior aspect of the wrist that becomes more prominent when the wrist is flexed and seems to diminish with wrist extension. What is the likely cause?

Ganglion cyst; they are filled with mucin and communicate with the adjacent joint space, tendon and/or tendon sheath via a stalk.

Surgery/Emergency Care

14. In the postoperative period, what is the most common cause of fever?

Wound infection (not atelectasis)

15. A patient falls on an outstretched hand and complains of wrist/base of thumb pain. The patient has tenderness within the anatomic snuff box, but the x-ray is read as normal. What do you do?

If no fracture is seen, scaphoid fracture cannot be ruled out. Repeat x-rays (including scaphoid views) should be obtained in 7–10 days. If negative and patient still has symptoms, obtain an MRI or bone scan.

16. In wrist pain, tenderness in the anatomical snuffbox is associated with fracture of what bone?

Scaphoid (only 40% specific)

17. What is the likely diagnosis in a patient with gum erythema, swelling, tenderness to touch, and edema? The gums bleed with brushing, flossing, or eating.

Acute gingivitis; often due to poor dental hygiene (secondary to plaque buildup). It is treated with chlorhexidine rinses, oral antibiotics (penicillins, metronidazole, doxycycline) and close follow-up with a dentist.

18. How should the presence of an incidentally found thyroid nodule be evaluated?

A TSH should be done; if normal, an ultrasound of the thyroid should be obtained, followed by radionuclide scan (scintigraphy). If "hot," no need for fine needle aspiration (FNA); if "cold" or patient is at high risk, do FNA.

19. What tendons are involved in de Quervain tenosynovitis?

De Quervain tenosynovitis is an overuse injury of the wrist that involves abductor pollicis longus and extensor pollicis brevis tendons.

20. What physical examination is used to diagnose de Quervain tenosynovitis?

De Quervain tenosynovitis is diagnosed by Finkelstein test (pain reproduced with folding the fingers over the thumb and passively deviating the thumb in an ulnar direction).

21. In patients with acute onset right lower quadrant (RLQ) abdominal pain, what is the test of choice for diagnosing acute appendicitis?

Computed tomography (CT) scan

22. Not long after starting a thiazide diuretic, a patient develops a painful, swollen, and erythematous knee without history of trauma; what is the likely diagnosis?

Gout often presents as an acute arthritis that can occur in the first metatarsophalangeal joint, mid-tarsal, ankle and knee joints. It is due to the deposition of monosodium urate (MSU) crystals that accumulate in joints and soft tissues resulting in acute and chronic arthritis, soft-tissue masses called tophi, urate nephropathy, and uric acid nephrolithiasis.

23. What is the most sensitive method to determine a patient's risk for postoperative bleeding?

A history of prior bleeding problems; not a laboratory evaluation

24. How should hands that are soiled or contaminated with blood or bodily fluids be cleaned?

Hands should be initially washed using soap and water.

25. Abdominal pain that seems out of proportion to findings on physical examination should suggest what condition?

Acute mesenteric ischemia

26. What percentage of patients with incidentally found gallstones will ultimately need surgery?

Approximately 20% will progress to symptomatic disease requiring surgery.

27. What is the implication on foot examination of slow (>2 seconds) capillary refill, thickened nails, and absence of hair on the toes?

Lower extremity arterial insufficiency

28. What vitamin deficiencies are caused by gastric bypass?

Vitamin B_{12}, iron, calcium, and vitamin D

29. What should be done in a patient with right upper quadrant (RUQ) abdominal pain consistent with biliary colic and a normal abdominal ultrasound?

A nuclear HIDA scan to identify acalculous cholelithiasis

30. What areas of the body are common locations for superficial spreading malignant melanoma by gender?

Upper back for both men and women; lower extremities for women

31. A skier goes to a mountain at 13,000 feet but becomes ill with a headache and nausea. What is the likely cause?

Acute mountain sickness, a form of high altitude sickness presents at over 8,000 feet of altitude (22% at 8,000; over 40% at 10,000), most often with headache and at least one of the following: Nausea/vomiting, fatigue/lassitude, dizziness, and/or difficulty sleeping. Symptoms begin 4–12 hours after ascent. For most, the symptoms are benign and self-limited.

32. What is the diagnostic test for pulmonary embolism?

CT pulmonary angiography

33. In what conditions should bilevel positive airway pressure (BiPAP) be deleterious?

Respiratory failure associated with sepsis, pneumonia, acute respiratory distress syndrome, or pneumothorax

34. For acute dental infections, what is the antibiotic of choice?	Oral penicillin G
35. A young male presents with acute right-sided chest pain; what test should be done to rule out spontaneous pneumothorax?	Chest x-ray
36. In an acute epistaxis, what blood vessels are the most common cause?	Kiesselbach plexus located on the anteroinferior septum
37. What component of blood is affected by aspirin ingestion?	Platelets are inhibited by aspirin.
38. In what condition is BiPAP primarily used?	BiPAP is commonly used in chronic obstructive pulmonary disease (COPD). This addresses the progressive respiratory acidosis with impending respiratory failure or fatigue. BiPAP improves ventilation while decreasing PCO_2 levels.
39. A patient complains of recurrent mid chest pain after eating. What condition is suggested by a dilated esophagus and an air-fluid level on chest x-ray?	Achalasia
40. A 17-year-old female has a syncopal event after sprinting in a race. At the ED, her ECG demonstrated a prolonged QT interval. What are the dangers of long QT syndrome?	Long QT syndrome is due to a prolonged QTc and may precipitate polymorphic ventricular tachycardia (VT) (torsade de pointes), leading to dizziness, syncope, and sudden cardiac death from ventricular fibrillation (VF). Common causes for ventricular fibrillation include emotional stress, sudden exertion, and certain medications.

Surgery/Emergency Care

41. What mechanism of injury causes radial head subluxation (nursemaid's elbow) in a child?	Sudden traction of an extended arm
42. How is radial head subluxation (nursemaid's elbow) treated?	Grasp hand in handshake position; stabilize radial head with the other hand with the thumb over the radial head; in fluid motion, first supinate forearm then flex elbow
43. What is the most common bacterial cause of community-acquired bacterial pneumonia in adults?	*Streptococcus pneumoniae*
44. What is the causative agent in bacterial meningitis in college students?	*Neisseria meningitidis*
45. What is spondylolysis?	Spondylolysis (defect or fracture within the pars interarticularis of the vertebral arch in the spinal column)
46. A 27-year-old male who was recently started on olanzapine for bipolar disorder presents to the ED with high fever and confusion associated with muscle rigidity; what is the likely cause?	Neuroleptic malignant syndrome often presents within a few weeks of starting an offending medication (typically antipsychotics) with symptoms of fever, muscular rigidity, altered mental status, and autonomic dysfunction.
47. What is spondylolisthesis?	Spondylolisthesis is the forward displacement of a vertebra, especially the fifth lumbar vertebra over S1, often due to a birth defect of the spine or acute trauma.
48. How long may scaphoid fractures take before they are visible on radiographs?	2 weeks (up to 20% of x-rays will be falsely negative at the time of injury)

Surgery/Emergency Care

49. Which structure is damaged in gamekeeper's (or Skier) thumb?

The condition is an avulsion of the ulnar collateral ligament (UCL) where the ligament is torn at the proximal MCP of the thumb, either from a fall/trauma (Skier's) causing an avulsion or chronic abduction (gamekeeper's) causing lengthening of the UCL.

50. Button battery ingestion in children should include what management?

If visible on x-ray in the esophagus, remove by immediate endoscopy. If it has passed into the stomach and either remains there more than 48 hours or the battery is larger than 2 cm in diameter, it should be removed endoscopically. If it has entered the duodenum, x-rays should be followed with expected expulsion within 72 hours.

51. A patient with multiple sclerosis (MS) develops loss of vision over the course of a few days; what is the diagnosis?

Optic neuritis can develop for many reasons, but patients with MS are a higher risk. Symptoms include brow ache, globe tenderness, and deep orbital pain exacerbated by eye movement. Intravenous (IV) steroids are the treatment of choice; using oral steroids may increase the risk of recurrence.

52. At what age would the presence of an undescended testicle prompt surgical evaluation?

6 months; surgery should be performed before 1 year of age. Surgery lowers risk of torsion and potential infertility, and lowers, but does not eliminate, risk of malignancy

53. In patients with type 2 diabetes with hyperosmolar hyperglycemia, what is the initial treatment?

Intravenous fluids and insulin administration

54. What is the most common site for diabetic patients to develop osteomyelitis?

The foot

55. Which population has the greatest risk of developing melanoma?

Men over age 50

56. What is paraphimosis?

Entrapment of the retracted foreskin; it is a medical emergency. Initial treatment includes applying ice to the region; definitive care involves a penile block followed by manual reduction.

57. What is the most common component of gallstones?

Cholesterol

58. What is the most common component of renal stones?

Calcium oxalate

59. Increased urine acidity is associated with what type of stone?

Uric acid stones; treatment involves alkalinizing the urine.

60. In a patient with recent head trauma, the finding of an air-fluid level in the sphenoid sinus should raise suspicion of what condition?

Basilar skull fracture

61. In a patient with head trauma, double vision and fluid in the maxillary sinus are associated with what condition?

Orbital floor fracture

62. What clinical findings and nerve distribution are involved in carpal tunnel syndrome?

Median nerve (palmar side of the thumb, the index and middle finger, and radial half of the ring finger)

Surgery/Emergency Care

63. What condition should be considered in a patient who has just returned from a recent scuba diving trip with fatigue, anorexia, headache, and loss of sensation in the trunk area and lower extremities?

Decompression illness (the "bends")

---

64. What is the test of choice for the detection of symptomatic renal stones?

Unenhanced helical CT scan of the abdomen and pelvis; it is better than ultrasound.

---

65. A few weeks following a viral infection, a patient presents with fatigue and hypotension; BP is 70/50 and heart sounds are muffled, with a friction rub. What is the most worrisome cause?

Post viral pericarditis that has induced a cardiac tamponade.

---

66. A patient presenting with no history of trauma but with a "patch of blood" under the conjunctiva on the inferior aspect of the eye has what condition?

Subconjunctival hemorrhage; observation is the only treatment

---

67. What rare condition is associated with an acute sphenoidal or ethmoidal sinusitis?

Cavernous sinus thrombosis

---

68. What is the protocol for postexposure rabies prophylaxis for a dog bite if the dog cannot be observed?

Rabies immune globulin followed by human diploid cell rabies vaccine

Surgery/Emergency Care

69. How is a pet hamster bite treated to prevent rabies?

Reassurance; bites from rabbits, squirrels, hamsters, guinea pigs, gerbils, chipmunks, rats, and mice almost never require antirabies treatment

70. A 31-year-old female presents with daily episodes of recurrent vomiting. She assures you she is not bulimic, but does state she uses marijuana on a daily basis. What is the likely diagnosis?

Cyclic vomiting syndrome; chronic, idiopathic disorder characterized by recurrent, discrete episodes of disabling nausea and vomiting separated by symptom-free intervals lasting a few days to months. Chronic marijuana use is a common etiology.

71. When a patient presents with multiple injuries in varying stages of healing, what diagnosis should be considered?

Physical abuse

72. What is the normal range of the ankle-brachial index?

0.9–1.00 (ankle systolic pressure at rest is normally 90% of the brachial systolic pressure); <0.9 or above 1.4 is considered abnormal

73. What clinical conditions should prompt an extensive evaluation when a DVT is diagnosed?

Age <50 with an idiopathic DVT, patients with recurrent DVT or pulmonary embolism, or patients with a family history of thromboembolism

74. What scuba diving injury is common?

Barotrauma; when gas-filled space does not equalize its pressure with external pressure; sinuses, inner, middle and external ear, GI tract, lungs, etc., are all at risk.

Surgery/Emergency Care

75. What type of arthropod can cause a bite that is initially a sharp pinprick sensation followed by resolution of the pain but systemic symptoms of cramping abdominal pain, muscle rigidity, sweating, nausea, vomiting, and shortness of breath?

Black widow spider envenomation

76. What medication is the most potent and effective treatment for an acute asthma attack?

Corticosteroids

77. When treating an acute asthmatic attack, what medications should be used as first-line therapy?

Short-acting β_2-agonists, and systemic steroids; antibiotics are not indicated unless a bacterial infection is suspected.

78. What are the benefits of inhaled corticosteroids over oral steroids for the maintenance and control of asthma?

Inhaled corticosteroids have fewer systemic side effects like osteoporosis, cataracts, and adrenal insufficiency.

79. Eye pain and photophobia are usually suggestive of what serious eye disorders?

Uveitis, keratitis, acute glaucoma, and orbital cellulitis

80. What is the diagnosis when a patient has recurrent and severe spasm-like pain in the rectum?

Proctalgia fugax

81. What is the most common diagnosis of a postmenopausal female with recurrent dysuria symptoms, blood on urinalysis, but negative urine cultures?

Interstitial cystitis

82. What is the underlying condition when a patient presents with a shoulder pain with active and passive range of motion (frozen shoulder or adhesive capsulitis)?

Impingement syndrome of the rotator cuff

83. What physical examinations are used to evaluate the integrity of the anterior cruciate ligament (ACL)?

Lachman test (knee is placed in 20 degrees of flexion and tibia is pulled anteriorly on a secured femur); a positive test result is indicated by increased tibial movement compared with the unaffected knee. The anterior draw test is slightly less sensitive, but easier to perform (knee flexed to 90 degrees and hip flexed to 45 degrees, interlock fingers behind the knee, using index fingers to assure hamstring relaxation). When pulling interiorly, extended translation of the tibia implies ACL tear.

84. What is the treatment of choice for a patient who presents with pilonidal abscess?

Incision and drainage; ultimately evaluation for communicating sinus tracts

85. What treatable condition is the most common cause for liver failure and transplantation in the United States?

Hepatitis C infection

86. After a cardiac event, how long do cardiac troponins remain elevated?

Cardiac troponins may remain elevated for 2 weeks after an event.

87. What noncardiac conditions may cause elevated troponin T levels?

Renal disease, polymyositis, or dermatomyositis

88. Olecranon bursitis typically is due to what etiology?

Repeated trauma to the elbow

89. What condition is associated with inflammation of the tendon sheath of the abductor pollicis longus and the extensor pollicis brevis?

De Quervain tenosynovitis

90. A urine dipstick that is positive for hemoglobin but has no erythrocytes on microscopic examination is suggestive of what condition?

Rhabdomyolysis with myoglobinuria

91. What are three hallmark symptoms in a patient with aortic stenosis?

Chest pain (angina), shortness of breath (dyspnea), and syncope

92. What is the clinical and treatment difference between heat stroke and heat exhaustion?

Heat stroke is a medical emergency; the body temperature is usually greater than 40°C and sweating is usually absent; with heat exhaustion, there is profuse sweating and the body temperature does not exceed 40°C.

93. A positive heterophile antibody test (monospot) is indicative of what infection?

Mononucleosis

94. What clinical finding in mononucleosis may limit sports participation?

Splenomegaly; can last up to 6–8 weeks

95. What disease is the most common cause of superior vena cava syndrome?

Carcinoma of the lung (especially small cell and squamous cell carcinoma)

96. What are the key ECG findings seen in atrial fibrillation?

Absence of P waves and irregular ventricular rhythm. The atrial rate can range from 400 to 600 bpm, whereas the ventricular rate usually ranges from 80 to 180 bpm in the untreated state.

97. What are the drugs of choice for patients with heart failure?

Angiotensin-converting enzyme inhibitor, β-blockers, if New York Heart Association class III or IV, aldosterone antagonists

98. Recurrent hyperextension of the first toe that results in inflammation of the first metatarsophalangeal joint is called?

Turf toe

99. What classes of antibiotics are commonly correlated with the development of *Clostridium difficile* colitis?

Penicillins, cephalosporins, and quinolones

100. Atraumatic pain with abduction of the shoulder above 90 degrees is suggestive of what condition?

Rotator cuff tendonitis (impingement syndrome)

101. Blunt foreign bodies can be observed in the esophagus for how long before endoscopic removal?

24 hours

102. What is the appropriate treatment of a needle-stick injury with a hollow bore needle that was used by an individual who is HIV negative?	Observation; copious irrigation; in cases where the exposure was from someone who is known to be HIV negative, no HIV prophylaxis is needed
103. What common agents may result in false-positive urine drug screens?	Poppy seeds, Vicks inhalers, selegiline, non-steroidal antiinflammatory drugs, rifampin, venlafaxine, dextromethorphan, oxaprozin, and fluoroquinolones
104. What is the most common cause of death immediately following bariatric surgery?	Pulmonary embolism
105. What are the body mass index (BMI) requirements for consideration of bariatric surgery in a type 2 diabetic?	In a Type 2 diabetic, bariatric (now called metabolic) surgery should be considered for a BMI of 40 kg/m^2 or greater, OR a BMI of greater than 30 kg/m^2 in a type 2 diabetic with poorly controlled disease
106. What electrolyte imbalance results with excessive vomiting?	Hypokalemia, hypochloremia, metabolic alkalosis
107. What test can help differentiate congestive heart failure (CHF) and COPD in acute dyspnea?	B-type natriuretic peptide (BNP); a BNP > 400 pg/mL has a high likelihood of CHF
108. Individuals with acute onset worrisome chest pain and multiple cardiac risk factors benefit from what diagnostic procedure?	Cardiac catheterization

109. In a patient with chest pain and has intermediate CV risk who is able to exercise and has a normal ECG, what is the diagnostic test of choice?

Treadmill exercise test

110. What test should be considered in a patient with acute chest pain who is at intermediate risk of IHD and has an abnormal ECG (left bundle branch block, early repolarization, left ventricular hypertrophy, or digoxin use)?

Nuclear stress test or stress echocardiogram

111. Knee pain that affects a quarter-sized area 2–6 cm below the medial joint line of the knee is likely what condition?

Pes anserine bursitis

112. What are the most common infectious agents in acute epididymitis in men under age 35 years?

Chlamydia trachomatis or *Neisseria gonorrhoeae*

113. In patients with what allergy history is influenza vaccine contraindicated?

Allergy to eggs

114. What antiviral agents are effective for both influenza A and B?

Zanamivir (Relenza) and oseltamivir (Tamiflu)

115. What is the most common infectious agent in acute epididymitis in men over age 35?

Coliform bacteria (i.e., *Escherichia coli*)

116. What is the diagnostic test of choice to rule out acute testicular torsion?	Testicular ultrasound
117. What is the most common cause of acute thyroid pain and tenderness?	Subacute thyroiditis usually related to a viral infection
118. When is antibiotic therapy appropriate in the treatment of bacterial rhinosinusitis?	Only if symptoms have not improved after 10 days or if they worsen after 5–7 days

119. On diagnostic paracentesis, what condition is consistent with ascitic fluid WBC count ≥500/mm³ with 50% polymorphonuclear leukocytes?	Acute bacterial peritonitis:
	    WBC count ≥500/mm³ with at least 50% being PMNs,
	    Protein count of >1 g/dL,
	    Glucose < 50 mg/dL,
	    LDH > 225 U/L

120. What class of drugs is indicated for the treatment of status epilepticus?	Benzodiazepines
121. A fracture of the proximal fifth metatarsal (Jones fracture) can be complicated by what condition?	Delayed union or nonunion
122. In postoperative care, what is the major advantage of patient-controlled anesthesia (PCA)?	Avoidance of oversedation
123. What are risk factors for drowning or near-drowning?	Male, between 1 and 5 years of age, low socioeconomic status, alcohol use

Surgery/Emergency Care

124. What class of pain medication causes spasm of the sphincter of Oddi?

All opioid analgesics, including meperidine

125. What narcotic pain medication has a neurotoxic metabolite that has the potential to accumulate and cause seizures, myoclonus, and tremors?

Meperidine (Demerol)

126. What blood products are used in treating low fibrinogen levels and factor deficiencies such as hemophilia A and von Willebrand disease?

Cryoprecipitate

127. Following acute head trauma, what test is used to detect a subdural hematoma?

Noncontrast CT

128. What is the common cause of hot tub folliculitis?

Pseudomonas aeruginosa

129. How much lung volume, in percent, can be treated with just observation in a spontaneous pneumothorax?

Up to 15%–20% of lung volume

130. What emergency intervention is used to treat a tension pneumothorax?

Decompression with a large bore needle placed in the second intercostal space

131. What high school sport is most commonly associated with concussion (traumatic brain injury)?

Football

132. What nerve is compromised in carpal tunnel syndrome?	Median nerve
133. In a newborn, what does a "double bubble" sign imply?	High or duodenal obstruction, including volvulus
134. A patient presents after falling and hitting the head. What are the signs and symptoms of a concussion?	<ul><li>Confusion</li><li>Posttraumatic (antegrade) amnesia</li><li>Retrograde amnesia</li><li>Loss of consciousness (occurs in <10%)</li><li>Disorientation</li><li>Feeling "in a fog," "zoned out"</li><li>Inability to focus (i.e., difficulty at work or school)</li><li>Delayed verbal and motor responses</li><li>Slurred/incoherent speech</li><li>Excessive drowsiness</li></ul>
135. In a patient with acute abdominal pain, a positive psoas sign (pain with passive extension of the hip) and obturator sign (pain with internal and external rotation of the flexed hip) suggest what diagnosis?	Acute appendicitis
136. What abnormal growth in the middle ear is associated with chronic otitis media, bony destruction, and perforation of the tympanic membrane?	Cholesteatoma, which is the formation of a squamous epithelial-lined sac in the middle ear
137. For an uncomplicated laceration, how long should facial sutures be placed before removal?	3–5 days

138. How long should sutures in areas subject to high tension be left in place?

10–14 days

139. In a patient with blunt chest trauma, what radiographic test can be initially used to detect esophageal rupture (Boerhaave syndrome)?

Chest radiograph

140. What classification of colon polyps are considered precancerous?

Villous adenomas

141. What malignancy risk is increased in someone with a history of Peutz-Jeghers syndrome?

Colon cancer

142. What clinical condition must be present to justify joint replacement surgery?

Intractable pain that does not respond to other medical treatment

143. What type of malignant melanoma is most common?

Superficial spreading type

144. What medication is used for life-threatening anaphylaxis?

Epinephrine

145. Which type of melanoma has the poorest prognosis?

Nodular melanoma; these lesions tend to spread deeply into the underlying tissue.

146. What blood type is the universal donor?

O-negative blood

147. A fall on to an outstretched hand can cause injury to what complex?	Triangular fibrocartilage complex
148. What is the current length of anticoagulation recommendations for an uncomplicated DVT of the calf?	3 months
149. Following an initial immunization series through teenage years, how frequently should adults be immunized for tetanus prevention?	Every 10 years
150. What blood pressure readings make a hypertensive crisis?	SBP > 179 mm Hg or a DBP > 109 mm Hg
151. What are the treatment goals for a hypertensive crisis?	Goal: MAP lowered by maximally 20% or to DBP 100–110 mm Hg within first hour, then gradual reduction in BP to normal over next 48–72 hours Drug of choice: nicardipine, clevidipine, or labetalol
152. What dose, in mg/kg, is considered toxic in acetaminophen overdose?	>150 mg/kg acutely ingested
153. What agent is used for acute acetaminophen overdose?	Administer *N*-acetylcysteine (NAC) based upon Rumack-Matthew nomogram. NAC is virtually 100% hepatoprotective if initiated within 8 hours of an acute overdose.
154. What arrhythmia is caused by a lightning strike?	Asystole; high-voltage alternating current may cause ventricular fibrillation.

Surgery/Emergency Care

155. Who should be screened for an abdominal aortic aneurysm (AAA)?

The USPSTF recommends one-time screening for AAA with ultrasonography in men ages 65–75 years who have ever smoked.

156. At what diameter should surgical repair of AAAs be offered?

5–6 cm (2005 ACC/AHA guidelines recommend repair when aneurysm is ≥5.5 cm.)

157. What is the difference between Stage 1 and Stage 2 decubitus ulcer?

Stage 1: Nonblanchable erythema of intact skin
Stage 2: Partial-thickness dermal or epidermal skin loss causing a blister, shallow crater, or abrasion

158. What is the difference between a Stage 3 and Stage 4 decubitus ulcer?

Stage 3: Full-thickness necrosis causing a deep crater down to the fascia
Stage 4: Full-thickness destruction of muscle, bone, or supporting structures

159. A smoker has a raised white plaque on the buccal mucosa; what is the likely diagnosis?

Leukoplakia

160. What is the risk of leukoplakia becoming cancerous?

Leukoplakia is benign. It is biopsied to confirm diagnosis, and can be used to encourage smoking cessation.

161. Which local anesthetic has the longest duration of action?

Bupivacaine

162. What locations should be avoided when injecting lidocaine with epinephrine?

Fingers, nose, penis, or toes (and ears)

163. What topical agents may be used to treat chronic anal fissures?

Topical nifedipine with lidocaine gel

Surgery/Emergency Care

164. A newborn who develops pneumonia in the lower segments of the upper lobes should be evaluated for what condition?	Tracheoesophageal fistula
165. What are the clinical indications for Mohs surgery?	A patient with a nonmelanoma skin cancer measuring >2 cm, lesions with indistinct margins, recurrent lesions, and lesions close to important structures including the eyes, nose, and mouth
166. At what level does lumbar disc disease occur?	L5–S1 interspace
167. Following hip surgery, how long should DVT anticoagulation prophylaxis be continued?	At least 10–14 days postoperatively; some data suggest up to 35 days
168. What size and location of kidney stone is best suited for treatment with lithotripsy?	If renal, <2 cm; if ureteral, <1 cm
169. When should a preoperative antibiotic be administered?	Within 60 minutes of incision
170. While playing basketball, a patient pivots off the knee, hears a loud "pop," and develops immediate pain and swelling. What is the likely diagnosis?	Acute ACL injury and tear
171. In what location do Morton neuromas arise?	The second and third interdigital space
172. What tendon injury results in a mallet finger?	An injury to the extensor tendon at the DIP joint

Surgery/Emergency Care

173. What tendon is injured in patients with a jersey finger?

Disruption of the flexor digitorum profundus tendon usually affecting the ring finger (75% of cases)

174. What are the physiologic benefits of suturing?

Suturing approximates the skin and eliminates unnecessary dead space; tension is be minimized.

175. What animal bites require rabies postexposure prophylaxis?

Bats, skunks, foxes, raccoons, and dogs (carnivores). You rarely need rabies prophylaxis for squirrels, hamsters, rabbits, gerbils, chipmunks, rats, or mice

176. In a hypotensive patient, what is the drug of choice for bradycardia?

Atropine

177. What class of drug is the first-line treatment for isolated systolic hypertension in the elderly?

Thiazide diuretics

178. What drugs should be administered when first care is given to a patient with an unexplained altered mental status?

Administer naloxone, thiamine, and glucose

179. What are the most common foods to induce anaphylaxis in children?

Milk, egg, wheat, soy, and peanuts

180. If a patient on β-blockers develops anaphylaxis, epinephrine may be less effective; what drug should be used to treat anaphylaxis in these patients?

Glucagon

181. What decision rule should be used to evaluate if an acute ankle sprain needs imaging?

The Ottawa Ankle Rules suggest that foot or ankle radiographs are unnecessary except when any of the following are present:
- Bony tenderness at the posterior edge of the distal 6 cm of the tibia or tip of either malleolus
- Bony tenderness along the base of the 5th metatarsal or navicular bone
- Inability to take four unassisted steps both immediately after the injury and in the ED

182. Treatment for mild to moderate ankle sprains should involve what sort of support?

Elastic bandage dressing coupled with an air stirrup splint

183. What is the most common cause of chronic ankle pain?

Incomplete rehabilitation of an acute ankle sprain; physical therapy involving proprioception and strength training will often resolve.

184. Organophosphate overdose is most commonly caused by what agents?

Pesticides

185. What are the symptoms of organophosphate poisoning?

Organophosphates deactivate cholinesterases, resulting in excess acetylcholine. Symptoms include the following:
- DUMBELS:
  - Diarrhea/diaphoresis
  - Urination
  - Miosis/muscle fasciculations
  - Bradycardia, bronchorrhea, bronchospasm
  - Emesis
  - Lacrimation
  - Salivation
- May have garlic odor

186. An elderly patient presents with atraumatic joint pain, swelling, warmth, and decreased range of motion. What is the most important diagnosis to rule out?

Septic joint

187. What is sudden onset unilateral loss of CN VII motor function (flaccid paralysis of facial muscles, including forehead) called?

Bell palsy

188. Bell palsy is often induced by

Reactivation of latent herpesvirus, Lyme disease, atherosclerosis, diabetes, any recent viral infection, hypertension

189. What bacterium is of concern in dog and cat bites?

Pasteurella multocida

190. What is the antibiotic of choice for animal bites?

Amoxicillin–clavulanic acid

191. In diabetic ketoacidosis (DKA), what are the mainstays of initial treatment?

IV hydration (1–2 L of NS over 1st hour)
IV insulin
Electrolyte correction

192. What percentage of women in the ED are there due to a domestic violence–related injury?

14%–35%

193. What is the cause of a bilateral facial erythematous rash that is associated with fever, often after a facial trauma?

Erysipelas is a distinct form of cellulitis notable for acute, well-demarcated, superficial bacterial skin infection with lymphatic involvement usually caused by *Streptococcus pyogenes*.

194. What is the difference between periorbital cellulitis and orbital cellulitis?

Periorbital cellulitis is an acute bacterial infection of the skin and tissue anterior to the orbital septum; it does not involve orbital structures (globe, fat, and ocular muscles).

Orbital cellulitis is acute infection of orbital contents posterior to orbital septum; it results in decreased eye ROM because of infection.

195. A patient presents with 2 weeks of chronic nonbloody diarrhea, but no other systemic symptoms. A wilderness camping trip a few weeks prior to the diarrhea onset is reported. What is the likely diagnosis?

Giardiasis

196. What is the treatment of choice for giardiasis?

Metronidazole 250 mg PO TID for 5–7 days

197. An elderly patient has a painful erythematous rash that follows a dermatomal distribution across the chest; you diagnose herpes zoster. What medications should be started within 72 hours of the rash's emergence?

Oral antivirals should be started within 72 hours of skin lesion onset. Corticosteroids are NO LONGER used, as they do not decrease the risk of postherpetic neuralgia.

198. A patient presents with a unilateral drooping eyelid; on examination, you notice the pupil on that side is smaller than the opposite side. What is the syndrome?

Horner syndrome presents as a classic triad of ipsilateral miosis, eyelid ptosis, and/or anhidrosis of the face and neck.

199. Smokers who develop Horner syndrome should be tested for what tumor?

Smokers with Horner syndrome need to have a Pancoast tumor of the lung ruled out with at least a chest x-ray.

200. An older patient has progressive lethargy, severe dehydration, electrolyte abnormalities, and a nonfasting glucose of >600 mg/dL but no ketones; what is the likely diagnosis?

Hyperosmolar hyperglycemic state; patient has undiagnosed type 2 diabetes mellitus with an insulin deficit. The resulting hyperglycemia acts as an osmotic diuretic, causing dehydration, an elevated serum osmolality, and relative hypernatremia (but no ketosis, as in DKA).

201. A patient is hit in the eye during a fight and now presents with slight blurring of vision and "blood in my eye." What is the diagnosis?

Hyphema; blood pools in anterior chamber (AC) of the eye (between iris and cornea), typically after some trauma to the region.

202. A parent presents with a child who has pustules on the face; after they rupture, the lesions develop a golden appearance. What is the diagnosis?

Impetigo, a contagious, superficial, intraepidermal infection occurring prominently on exposed areas of the face and extremities; etiology is often *Staphylococcus aureus* alone or in combination with Group A β-hemolytic strep.

203. What is the treatment of choice for mild to moderate impetigo?

Topical agents like mupirocin (Bactroban) 2% topical ointment or retapamulin 1% ointment; for more extensive infections, oral dicloxacillin may be used.

204. Which patients should be treated for acute influenza with oral antivirals?

Those who present within 48 hours of symptom onset AND those with comorbidities (infants, elderly, those with asthma, COPD, cardiovascular disease, diabetes, etc.); those without comorbidities should be treated symptomatically.

Surgery/Emergency Care

205. What condition is likely with sudden onset of vertigo (room spinning) when rolling over in bed or any change with regard to gravity that lasts for seconds to minutes?

Benign paroxysmal positional vertigo (BPPV) is a mechanical disorder of the inner ear characterized by a brief period of vertigo experienced when the position of the patient's head is changed relative to gravity.

206. What diagnostic maneuver is used to confirm the diagnosis of BPPV?

The Dix-Hallpike test (DHT) is used to diagnose BPPV. The patient is positioned in long-sitting on the exam table with the knees extended. If testing the right posterior canal, the head is rotated 45 degrees to the right. The patient is then lowered to supine position with the head 30–40 degrees below the horizontal, over the edge of the exam table for 45 seconds. *The physician observes the direction of the fast phase of the nystagmus.* The patient is then returned to the seated position, and the procedure is repeated toward the left.

207. How do you perform Epley maneuver in the treatment of BPPV?

Canalith repositioning procedure (CRP) or Epley maneuver is used to treat BPPV. The clinician moves the patient through four provoking positions. The head is rotated toward the right (uninvolved side). Maintaining this head rotation, the patient is rolled onto the right side (uninvolved side) with the head slightly elevated from the supporting surface. The patient then sits up and flexes the neck 36 degrees. Each position is maintained for a minimum of 45 seconds or as long as the nystagmus lasts. The procedure is repeated three times.

208. What conditions cause vertigo that lasts for hours or days?

TIA, stroke, seizures, new-onset multiple sclerosis, vestibular neuritis

209. What electrolyte in DKA often appears incorrectly lowered?

Sodium; DKA induces a dilutional pseudohyponatremia.

Surgery/Emergency Care

210. A breastfeeding mother is diagnosed with mastitis and placed on antibiotics. Can she continue to breastfeed?

Yes, mother and child are believed to be colonized with the same organism and the breast milk may be protective.

211. Patients who develop struvite renal stones commonly have what in their history?

Urinary tract infections with urea-splitting bacteria

212. What class of drugs increases the risk of floppy iris syndrome that can occur following cataract surgery?

Alpha antagonists, typically used to treat benign prostatic hypertrophy (BPH): alfuzosin (Uroxatral), doxazosin (Cardura), and tamsulosin (Flomax)

CHAPTER

6 Geriatrics

1. Urge incontinence (sudden onset of desire to urinate that results in incontinence before getting to restroom) results from which anatomic dysfunction?	Detrusor instability
2. What classes of medications increase the risk of falls in the elderly?	Sedative hypnotics, tricyclic antidepressants, neuroleptics, benzodiazepines, and Type IA antiarrhythmics
3. Lichen simplex chronicus in women is associated with what malignancy?	Vulvar carcinoma
4. What medications are useful in the treatment of pain because of compression fractures?	Analgesics, recombinant parathyroid hormone, calcitonin (injectable or intranasal), bisphosphonates, selective estrogen receptor modulators (SERMs)
5. What clinical findings are present in patients with Lewy body dementia?	Dementia Parkinsonism *Visual* hallucinations
6. The USPSTF recommends initiation of screening for osteoporosis at what age?	65 if no risk factors; 60–64 if risk factors are present
7. How is absorption altered in drug metabolism in elderly patients?	Absorption is slower, but generally as complete as in younger patients.

8. What form of abuse is the most common in the elderly?	Neglect; women are more affected than men.
9. What group of individuals are the most common perpetrators of abuse in the elderly?	Relatives of the abused (especially adult children)
10. What is the classic clinical triad of symptoms for normal pressure hydrocephalus (NPH)?	Ataxia Urinary incontinence Dementia (wet, wobbly, wacky)
11. What is the most common etiology of seizures in geriatric patients?	Cerebrovascular disease (especially hemorrhagic strokes)
12. In men with benign prostatic hyperplasia (BPH), how does finasteride and dutasteride affect prostate-specific antigen (PSA) levels?	They can reduce levels by half, making the detection of prostate cancer difficult; a baseline should be obtained before drug initiation, and follow-up testing should be interpreted recognizing this reduction
13. In the geriatric population, what is the most common cause of blindness?	Age-related macular degeneration
14. What are the clinical signs and symptoms of Parkinson disease?	Tremor at rest ("pill rolling") Bradykinesia (reduced arm swing when walking, micrographia) Rigidity (lead pipe or cogwheeling) Shuffling, festinating gait

15. With what disease a positive Babinski (upgoing toes after stroking lateral heel to metatarsal pad) sign is associated with?

Upper motor neuron and central disease, including multiple sclerosis, pernicious anemia, cerebral tumors, subdural hematoma, and spinal cord disease. It is *not* associated with Parkinson disease.

16. What is the initial drug of choice for treating Parkinson disease?

Levodopa

17. To qualify for hospice benefits, the patient must be judged to have how long of a life expectancy?

Less than 6 months for any diagnosis

18. Following breast cancer surgery, what routine surveillance is recommended?

Monthly breast self-examination
Annual mammography; history and physical examination every 6 months for the first 5 years and then annually
Routine surveillance with intensive laboratory and radiographic studies has *not* been shown to improve quality of life or survival

19. What are the initial treatment recommendations for urge incontinence?

Behavioral therapy with bladder training and pelvic floor muscle (Kegel) exercises; these are more effective than anticholinergic medication.

20. What class of medication is used for patients with excessive secretions at the end of life?

Anticholinergics (i.e., glycopyrrolate, scopolamine)

21. What are the treatment options for initial *Clostridium difficile* infection?

Oral metronidazole; treatment failure can be treated with another course of metronidazole or oral vancomycin. For recurrent or resistant *C. difficile*, fidaxomicin and fecal transplants are options.

22. Tuberculosis infection involving the bony spine is called:

Pott disease

Geriatrics

23. What type of incontinence is associated with a weak urinary sphincter and is associated with incontinence that occurs with coughing or sneezing?	Stress incontinence
24. What vitamin supplementation may decrease the risk of falls?	Vitamin D
25. What intervention can improve survival in patients with end-stage, severe COPD?	Oxygen
26. Screening tests are considered not beneficial if the patient's life expectancy is less than how many years?	10 years
27. Which class of antihypertensive agents will help preserve bone density?	Thiazide diuretics
28. In men, what are the risk factors for the development of osteoporosis?	Hypogonadism, corticosteroid use of >3 months, and vitamin D deficiency
29. What PSA velocity is predictive of prostate cancer?	0.75 ng/mL/yr
30. What is the risk of prostate cancer as the percentage of free PSA (unbound) goes up?	As the ratio of free (unbound) PSA goes up, the risk of prostate cancer goes down. When <10% of PSA is free, the positive predictive value for prostate cancer is 55%, when >25% of PSA is unbound, the risk is only 8%.

Geriatrics

31. What type of tremor may be reduced with the use of alcohol?	Essential tremor
32. A sudden loss of vision that is without pain suggests what diagnosis?	Retinal detachment
33. When a patient describes a "curtain or veil coming down" in their visual field suggests what diagnosis?	Retinal detachment
34. What blood tests should be done as part of the evaluation of restless leg syndrome (RLS)?	Hemoglobin, hematocrit, serum ferritin, and transferrin saturation—low ferritin and transferrin levels are associated with RLS.
35. What is the test used for assessing thyroid function in the elderly?	Thyroid-stimulating hormone
36. What condition is the leading risk factor for the development of delirium?	Dementia
37. What is the initial treatment of hypercalcemia associated with malignancy?	Aggressive rehydration and diuresis with furosemide; phosphorus replacement if hypophosphatemia is present, and administration of intravenous bisphosphonates.
38. What are the primary services offered by hospice?	Dietary counseling; short-term hospital and respite care, medication, and supplies to treat symptoms of terminal illness (but not medication used to cure the illness); physical, occupational, and speech therapies

Geriatrics

39. Megestrol acetate (Megace) acting as progestin agonist to improve appetite in those with cachexia has what side effects?

Thrombophlebitis, pulmonary embolism, and adrenal suppression (in high doses for prolonged periods)

40. When a patient has severe neuromuscular weakness, what procedure is used to prove myasthenia gravis?

The Tensilon test is used to diagnose myasthenia gravis.

41. Which SSRI has been used for the treatment of hot flash symptoms?

Paroxetine

42. What screening mammography testing interval does Medicare pay for?

Every 2 years

43. What is the best time to do breast self-examination in a premenopausal woman?

During the first week following menses

44. When treating Alzheimer dementia, what are the common side effects that result in the discontinuation of acetylcholinesterase inhibitors (tacrine, donepezil, rivastigmine, and galantamine)?

Gastrointestinal side effects including nausea, vomiting, and diarrhea

45. What areas are often cultured in methicillin-resistant *Staphylococcus aureus* (MRSA) colonization?

Nasal mucosa and oropharynx

Geriatrics

46. How is MRSA colonization treated to reduce the shedding of MRSA organisms?	Mupirocin (Bactroban)
47. Which flu symptom (fever, cough, sore throat, rhinorrhea, myalgias, headaches, fatigue) are less common in the elderly?	Fever
48. What is the most worrisome complication in the elderly when they develop influenza?	Pneumonia and associated respiratory decompensation
49. Unlike younger patients who develop chest pain, what symptoms do the elderly develop that represent their cardiac ischemia?	Dyspnea
50. A high-pitched, blowing diastolic murmur and a wide pulse pressure are suggestive of what diagnosis?	Aortic valve insufficiency
51. What is the life expectancy of symptomatic elderly patients with untreated aortic stenosis?	2–3 years
52. What clinical features discern delirium from dementia?	Time of symptoms; delirium has an acute onset and fluctuating course; dementia has a gradual, worsening course.
53. An acceleration–deceleration head injury can result in what sort of injury?	Subdural hematoma which results from tearing and rupture of the bridging veins beneath the dura

Geriatrics

54. A crescentic collection on CAT scan over one hemisphere of the brain that does not cross the midline is suggestive of what diagnosis?

Subdural hematoma

---

55. What initially differentiates Pick dementia from Alzheimer dementia?

Pick disease (frontotemporal dementia) is an inherited disorder that does NOT initially present with memory loss; it affects the frontal lobes and causes aphasia and behavioral problems. Alzheimer often presents initially with short-term memory loss.

---

56. Pick disease is inherited by what genetic-type pattern?

Autosomal-dominant inherited disease

---

57. What condition presents with loss of muscle strength and coordination, including difficulty opening and closing the jaw, drooling, voice change, hoarseness, muscle cramps, and stiffness and progresses to paralysis and death?

Amyotrophic lateral sclerosis, which affects both upper and lower motor neurons; sensory, cerebellar, and extraocular muscle functions are not affected.

---

58. What is the document used in nursing care facilities that represents a comprehensive resident assessment?

Minimum data set; it is required to detail patients' functional capacities.

---

59. What is the likely cause of loss of central vision, but intact peripheral vision?

Macular degeneration causes central vision to be lost, but peripheral vision usually remains intact.

Geriatrics

60. An elderly male presents with yellowish spots on fundoscopic exam; what is the cause?

Drusen which are fatty desposits under the retina that does not cause macular degeneration, but does increase the risk of developing macular degeneration

61. Which type of macular degeneration has the higher risk for loss of vision?

The exudative (or wet) form; the atrophic (or dry) form is usually less severe.

62. What condition results from decreased function of dopamine-containing neurons in the substantia nigra?

Parkinson disease

63. What are the clinical findings in a patient with Parkinson disease?

Bradykinesia; a pill-rolling tremor, cogwheel or lead pipe rigidity, infrequent blinking, blank stare, shuffling gait with a rapid initiation and the inability to stop once started (also called festinating gait), and increased salivation

64. Levodopa–carbidopa (Sinemet) should be taken with what kind of meal?

Low-protein meal; high-protein meals will decrease the bioavailability.

65. What is the rationale of using low dosages of levodopa and using short dosing intervals?

To prevent the "on–off effect" that is associated with fluctuations in the response to levodopa

66. What is the pathologic process of multiple sclerosis?

Autoimmune T cells cause damage in the white matter of the motor strip, causing symptoms of visual disturbances (extraocular eye muscle dysfunction, optic neuritis–induced unilateral blindness), decreased sensation, and coordination dysfunction.

Geriatrics

67. An elderly patient complains of sudden-onset need to urinate and of loss of urine before being able to reach bathroom. What is the likely diagnosis?

Urge incontinence; because of detrusor hyperactivity

68. Patients who state they loss their urine with cough or sneezing have what type of incontinence?

Stress incontinence; often due to pelvic floor relaxation

69. Patients with loss of urine without warning or without feelings of fullness, leakage of urine while sleeping, and an intermittent urinary stream have what type of incontinence?

Overflow incontinence

70. Which illnesses increase the risk of geriatric depression?

Stroke and cancer diagnoses are the two most highly correlated with the onset of depression.

71. What patient training should be given to treat chronic urinary incontinence?

Kegel exercises (repeated tightening and relaxation of the pelvic floor muscles)

72. What social condition increases the risk of geriatric depression?

Social isolation

73. Vaginal pruritus, burning, discharge, and excessive dryness with dyspareunia are consistent with what diagnosis?

Atrophic vaginitis

Geriatrics

74. What topical agent is used first line to treat atrophic vaginitis?

Topical estrogen

75. What is the likely diagnosis in someone with new-onset dementia, gait ataxia, and urinary incontinence?

Normal pressure hydrocephalus

76. In men, what is the most common solid malignancy?

Prostate cancer

77. Following a radical prostatectomy, what are the most common complications?

Urinary incontinence and erectile dysfunction

78. What type of injury is associated with >10% risk of mortality in the geriatric population?

Hip fracture

79. After a fall, a senior citizen is found to have a leg that appears shortened, abducted, and externally rotated. What is the most likely diagnosis?

Hip fracture

80. With use of bisphosphonates, what is the most common adverse effect?

Gastrointestinal complaints including esophageal irritation

81. After falls, what is the second most common cause of trauma in senior citizens?

Motor vehicle accidents

Geriatrics

82. What is the likely cause of a patient who presents with numbness of the hands and feet, decreased taste, and swelling or soreness of the tongue?

B_{12} deficiency

83. What diabetic medication is not associated with hypoglycemia and considered safe if GFR is ≥30?

Metformin

84. What rare complication of metformin can occur if an elderly patient has a GFR <30 or acute renal failure?

Lactic acidosis

85. What class of medications is considered first line in the treatment of dementia?

Acetylcholinesterase inhibitors

86. Loss of short-term and recent memory and the presence of senile plaques, neurofibrillary tangles, and granulo-vacuolar degeneration of neurons is associated with what condition?

Alzheimer disease

87. During what rehabilitation time frame will most improvement be found following a stroke?

The first 12 weeks

Geriatrics

88. In a geriatric patient, what test of mobility and function can be used to detect an increased risk for falls?

The "get up and go" test. Patient is instructed to stand from a sitting position without using their hands, walk 10 feet, turn, and return to the chair to sit. Greater than 16 seconds to complete the process suggests postural instability or gait impairment.

89. Decreased visual acuity, noted primarily with reading and with decreased night vision and excessive glare in bright light or sunlight is associated with what diagnosis?

Cataracts

90. What time frame is used to define menopause?

The absence of menses for 6 months

91. What laboratory test can be used to detect menopause?

FSH ≥30 mIU/mL is consistent with ovarian failure.

92. What is a written advance directive that assigns one person as a decision-maker called?

Health care proxy

93. What is the term used for a written advance directive where a competent person indicates their medical preferences?

Living will

94. How does aging effect fasting glucose levels?

Increasing fasting blood glucose (1 mg/dL for every 10 years), although most remain within normal limits.

Geriatrics

95. A geriatric patient presents with visual hallucinations, memory loss, and some symptoms of Parkinson but no tremor; what is the likely diagnosis?	Lewy body dementia presents with dementia, delirium, and visual hallucinations with parkinsonism (use the acronym DDaVP); tremor is often absent.
96. What common drugs may induce a B_{12} deficiency?	Metformin and proton pump inhibitors (omeprazole, others) can induce a B_{12} deficiency; chronic alcohol use may as well.
97. How does aging effect fat-soluble medications?	As people age, their creatinine clearance increases and as does their body stores of fat. This leads to increased volume of distribution and longer half-life of fat-soluble medications in the body.
98. What are the indications for screening for an abdominal aortic aneurysm?	Men aged 65–75 who have ever smoked
99. How does aging effect creatinine clearance?	It decreases; normally a 10% decrease in creatinine clearance per 10 years after 40 years of age.
100. Hearing loss in the elderly is typically associated with loss of which frequencies?	High-frequency hearing loss, also called presbycusis
101. How is osteoporosis defined using a bone mineral density test?	A "T-score" greater than 2.5 standard deviations below the gender-adjusted mean for normal young adults at peak bone mass
102. How is osteopenia defined using a bone mineral density test?	A T score of −1.0 to −2.5

Geriatrics

103. At what age should an average risk woman be screened for osteoporosis?

At age 65 years; if she has multiple risk factors (low BMI, smoker, strong family history of early osteoporosis), at age 60 years

104. On bone mineral testing, what does the Z score mean?

It compares the patient's measurement with a population adjusted for age, gender, and race.

105. How often will Medicare pay for bone density examinations?

At age 65 for screening and then every 2 years for those undergoing treatment

106. How do thiazide diuretics affect bone density?

They decrease urinary excretion of calcium and improve bone density

107. What is the mechanism of action of raloxifene (Evista)?

It is an SERM (selective estrogen receptor modulator); it is indicated for both osteoporosis prevention and treatment and for breast cancer prevention

108. When used for BPH, why is tamsulosin (Flomax) preferred compared to other α-adrenergic antagonists?

It has a much lower risk of hypotension.

109. Why does tamsulosin (Flomax) not induce hypotension?

It is an $\alpha 1$ selective adrenoreceptor inhibitor, which is only found in the prostate.

110. What is the common cardiac concern in an elderly patient with hyperthyroidism?

Atrial fibrillation

111. What agents are available to treat a healthy 70-year-old who has an essential tremor?

β-Blockers are first line; if intolerant, consider primidone (Mysoline), an antiseizure medication, topiramate or gabapentin.

Geriatrics

112. What brief test can be used to screen for dementia?	Mini-Cog, which as three steps: first, ask the patient to repeat three random words, then draw a clock face set to "10 minutes to 2," and then recall the original three words. It is 99% sensitive and 93% specific for dementia.
113. In a 65-year-old woman with lower abdominal pain and a palpable ovary, what diagnosis is most concerning?	Ovarian cancer
114. What type of hypertension is more common and worrisome in elderly patients?	Systolic hypertension
115. What is the most common cause of injury-related emergency room visits in geriatric patients?	Falls
116. Geriatric men with untreated hypogonadism have a higher risk of what condition?	Osteoporosis
117. What population should be vaccinated for herpes zoster?	Age 60 years and older
118. What drugs are unsafe to use for chronic insomnia in the elderly?	Melatonin, benzodiazepines, and nonbenzodiazepine hypnotics are contraindicated as they are associated with an increased risk of falls, fractures, and death.
119. What condition is the leading cause of disability in patients over age 65?	Osteoarthritis

Geriatrics

120. Clinical symptoms of osteoarthritis include what findings?

Dysfunction and distortion of the distal interphalangeal joints (DIP) and proximal interphalangeal joints (PIP) joints of the fingers (but not the metacarpophalangeal joint [MCP] or wrist), lack of systemic findings, and minimal joint inflammation

121. A patient presents with "bumps" on the distal interphalangeal joints of her fingers associated with morning hand stiffness; what is the cause?

Heberden nodes form at the DIP joints in osteoarthritis.

122. What nonpharmacologic treatment should be initiated whenever treating lower extremity osteoarthritis?

Physical therapy with the goal of strength training (decreases pain) and endurance (aerobics, which improves long-term functionality). Benefits are lost within 6 months of exercise cessation.

123. How commonly do senior citizens live below the poverty level?

About 45% of US senior citizens live at or below the poverty level; seniors living alone or those over 80 have the greatest risk. Lack of adequate nutrition can be addressed by food stamps.

124. What is the risk of developing varicella zoster?

Approximately one in three seniors over 60 will develop shingles; that number approaches 50% before age 80.

125. What are the current pneumococcal vaccine recommendations for seniors?

Those 65 and older who have not received any pneumococcal vaccine should be given PCV 13 (Prevnar) first, followed by a dose of PPSV23 (Pneumovax) a year later.

126. For what diseases should all seniors be counseled to receive vaccines?

Influenza, shingles (herpes zoster), diphtheria, tetanus, pertussis (whooping cough), pneumococcal disease (pneumonia)

Geriatrics

127. A senior presents with a painful vesicular rash on his chest that starts under his axilla and extends anteriorly to the midclavicular line; what is the likely diagnosis?

Varicella zoster (shingles)

128. What rules can seniors follow to prevent (and initially treat) chronic constipation?

High-fiber diet, adequate fluids, exercise, and training to "obey the urge" to defecate (rectal distention initiates the defecation reflex; voluntarily overriding this reflex because of convenience or distraction is a common etiology)

129. What two commonly used medications increase the risk of chronic constipation?

Antacids (calcium, aluminum) and calcium channel blockers

130. In addition to increased exercise, increased fluid intake, and bowel training, what oral agents help treat chronic constipation?

Hydrophilic colloids (bulk-forming agents) like psyllium (konsyl, metamucil, perdiem fiber) and osmotic laxatives (polyethylene glycol, PEG) (MiraLax); all must be taken with adequate hydration or constipation may worsen

131. An elderly patient complains of her rhinorrhea whenever she eats; what is the likely diagnosis?

Gustatory rhinitis. Other types of nonallergic rhinitis in seniors include vasomotor and α-adrenergic hyperactivity (because of antihypertensives). All three can be treated with topic anticholinergic nasal spray (ipratropium); narrow-angle glaucoma is a relative contraindication to this drug.

132. A patient with history of smoking has worsening dyspnea; on spirometry, their forced expiratory velocity (FEV_1)/ forced vital capacity (FVC) is <0.7; what is the likely diagnosis?

Chronic obstructive pulmonary disease

Geriatrics

7 General Facts

1. Define sensitivity.	The percent of test results that are truly positive. True positives divided by the total number of positive results.
2. Define specificity.	The percent of test results that are truly negative. True negatives divided by the total number of negative results.
3. Define number needed to treat.	Number needed to treat (NNT) is the number of patients that need to be treated to prevent an outcome. It is 100 divided by the absolute difference between the percent in the intervention group minus the percent in the control group NNT = 100/ARR = [incidence in control group – incidence in treatment group]. E.g. If the absolute risk reduction (ARR) is 40% in control group and 20% in treated group, NNT = 100/(40 – 20) = 100/(20) = 5; you need to treat five people for the time period used in the study to get one occurrence of the outcome.
4. Define absolute risk reduction (ARR).	The absolute risk reduction is the absolute difference of the percent of an outcome in the control group minus the percent outcome in the intervention group. ARR = incidence (control group) – incidence (intervention group)
5. Define relative risk reduction (RRR).	The relative decrease of an outcome compared to the risk of that outcome in the control group. It is calculated by dividing the absolute risk reduction by the risk in the control group. RRR = (incidence [control group] – incidence [treated group])/incidence (control group)

6. Define *p* value.	The degree or limits of statistical significance. In medicine, a *p* value of <0.05 implies statistical significance (that the findings have a less than 5% chance of being incorrect).
7. Define confidence interval.	It is a measure of variance, predicting statistical significance. It is clinically similar to a *p* value, and notes the range of a measure where the actual number statistically lies.
8. What is the FDA's process to evaluate the safety and efficacy of new medications?	Phase 1: (Safety) a new medication is given to healthy adults to determine the drug's most common side effects and the drug's metabolism and excretion. Phase 2: (Efficacy) small study to determine if the drug shows benefit in patients who have a certain disease or condition. Phase 3: (Safety and efficacy) much larger scale trials in patients with a given disease but in conjunction with other medications to determine safety and efficacy. Phase 4: (Post marketing) after approval, the medication is further studied to determine more about long-term risks, optimal use, and efficacy in different populations.
9. What is primary prevention?	Primary prevention involves information or interventions directed toward the entire population. It includes health promotion (exercise, eat properly, etc.) and protection against exposures (wear seat belts, drink clean water) that can lead to health problems.
10. What is secondary prevention?	Measures taken based on potential risk factors like age or other objective measures (BMI, blood pressure, etc.). They are used early in the course of an illness to identify those who are affected but are without symptoms (screening for hypertension or colorectal cancer).

11. What is tertiary prevention?

Steps taken after the development of a condition that help rehabilitate patients by reducing complications, improving their quality of life, and extending their years of productivity (pneumococcal immunization after splenectomy, using statins post myocardial infarction [MI], etc.).

12. What is a systematic review?

A systematic review is a type of medical study that uses unbiased methods to find, evaluate, and combine outcomes of similar studies to determine if the combined data finds a different outcome than any one study.

Studies included in a systematic review are screened to include those of high quality and low risk of bias.

INDEX